*Dedicated to Dr Song X
and encou*

Contents

Image credits

Front cover: © imagewerks/Getty Images

Back cover: © Jakub Semeniuk/iStockphoto.com, © Royalty-Free/Corbis, © agencyby/iStockphoto.com, © Andy Cook/iStockphoto.com, © Christopher Ewing/iStockphoto.com, © zebicho – Fotolia.com, © Geoffrey Holman/iStockphoto.com, © Photodisc/Getty Images, © James C. Pruitt/iStockphoto.com, © Mohamed Saber – Fotolia.com

Meet the author

OM

Your interest in yoga is both inspiring and exciting. By way of introducing this book, I'd like to tell you a bit about my background and how I came to write the book.

I have been practising yoga for more than 40 years – and teaching it for about 35. Even as an experienced teacher, I continue to study. Several years ago, I took a sabbatical from teaching and writing to spend a year in the Himalayas, focusing on my personal practice. At that time, I became acutely aware of how some of the teachings of yoga might appear complex to the average Westerner.

Yoga is a vibrant, living tradition that has been passed down from teacher to student over thousands of years. It is the experience of unifying your individual soul with the Universal Soul. It is also the process by which you bring your mind to a state of absolute calmness so that this experience can take place.

The teachings of yoga often seem contradictory – little is black and/or white; much is poetic imagery. I observed how Western students and teachers of yoga, who cannot read Sanskrit and are not versed in Indian culture, literature, scriptures and mythology, often miss out on many important cultural references when they pick up a yoga book. I hope this book will enable you to understand the ancient teachings of yoga in ways that are relevant to your modern lifestyle.

May you have great success in your yoga practice. May you experience excellent health, long life and inner peace.

Swami Saradananda

Only got a minute?

One minute is enough time to calm your mind using a full breath (also see page 120).

▸ Sit in a comfortable position with your back straight and your eyes and mouth closed. Breathe gently through your nose.

▸ Feel the sensation of your breath as it flows softly in and out of your nostrils.

▸ Feel the beginning, the middle and the end of each in-breath. Watch how your lungs fill and your breath stops momentarily as it turns itself around to become your out-breath. Notice how the end of your out-breath stops slightly (retention of empty lungs) and then becomes your in-breath. As you observe the ongoing cycle of your breath, notice how your body and mind are becoming more relaxed.

- Your breath may be long or short; there is no need to change it. The important thing is to make your breath very regular – and to watch it.
- Become aware of the different qualities of your in-breath and your out-breath – also the qualities of the two pauses.
- If you find your attention shifting to an object other than your breath, gently but firmly remind yourself to bring your attention back to your breath.
- While you are following your breath you may become aware of various physical sensations in your body. This means that you no longer have your attention focused on your breath. Instead of berating yourself for not staying with your breath, imagine that you are breathing the sensation out with your next out-breath. Then gently but firmly bring your attention back to your breath.

5 Only got five minutes?

Five minutes is enough time for you to warm up and energize your body.

Tadasana: spend 30 seconds grounding yourself (see the picture on page 44).

1 Stand with your feet 2–3 inches (5–10 cm) apart and your knees straight. Ensure that your body weight is distributed evenly between your two feet.
2 Lift your toes and spread them wide apart as you replace them on the ground. Close your eyes and become aware of the exchange of energy between your feet and the earth. Visualize yourself sending roots down into the earth to draw its energy up into your body.
3 Feel the energy spreading upward into your legs. Feel your shins over your heels. Make sure that your knees are straight, but not locked.
4 As the energy comes into your trunk, ensure that your hips are straight. Imagine that you are bringing your tail bone forward to meet your pelvic bone.
5 Allow your arms to relax alongside your body, with your elbows straight but soft. Be sure that your chest is lifted, your spine erect, your shoulders relaxed. Feel as though your collar bones are broadening.
6 Keep your head upright. Gaze straight ahead, checking that your body remains straight.

Six sun salutations

(See the pictures on pages 30–33.)

1 Stand in tadasana. **Inhale deeply** and prepare yourself mentally to begin.

2 **Breathe out** as you bring your palms together directly in front of your breast bone. This classical hand position, known as 'namaskar', helps you to centre your body and mind.

3 **Breathe in** as you straighten your arms and stretch them up alongside your ears. Arch your entire body backwards, keeping your knees and elbows straight.

4 **Exhale** and bend forward. Place your hands on the ground on either side of your feet. Bring your head in towards your knees. If you have difficulty reaching the ground, allow your knees to bend slightly.

5 **Inhale** as you stretch your right leg back as far as possible. Bend both knees and place the back knee on the ground. Look up, keeping your hands on the ground on either side of your left foot.

6 **Hold your breath** as you bring your left foot back in line with your right; straighten both knees. Your body is now in a straight line from head to heels.

7 **Exhale** as you bend your knees and bring them directly downwards to the ground. Keep your hips up and drop your chest to the ground between your hands. Place your chin on the ground.

8 Without moving your hands or your feet, **inhale** as you slide your body forward and arch into the cobra pose. Keep your abdomen on the ground. Your elbows are bent slightly and in towards your sides. Your shoulders are relaxed and down, away from your ears.

9 Tuck your toes under and **breathe out** as you lift your hips high. Straighten your elbows and allow your head to hang down between your arms. Bring your chest closer to your thighs; stretch your heels to the ground.

10 **Inhale**; bend your left knee and place it down to the ground. Step forward with your right foot. Make sure that your toes are in line with your fingers. Look up without lifting your hands off the ground.

11 Bring your left foot forward, next to your right; **exhale**. Lift your hips up and drop your head down towards your knees. Straighten your knees as much as possible, without lifting your hands off the ground.

12 **Inhale** as you slowly straighten your body; stretch your arms forward and then up over your head. Arch back into the same position as you were in step 3.

13 **Exhale** as you lower your arms by your sides and return to tadasana.

In the first sun salutation, you lead with your right foot. In the next one, you lead with your left foot.

Standing crescent moon

Beginning in Tadasana (again, see the picture on page 44).

1 **Inhale** as you raise your arms straight out to the sides and then over your head in a lateral, circular motion. When your hands meet, interlock your fingers. Release your index fingers so that they are pointing upward. Keep your elbows straight. Stretch your entire body upwards.

2 Keeping this stretch, **exhale** as you arch your torso to the right as much as possible. Do not allow your body to twist.

3 **Inhale** as you return to centre.

Repeat this on your left side.

This is the beginning of the moon salutation. If you have time, you may want to do the full sequence; the instructions are on pages 34–41.

Lie down and relax for at least a minute before you leave your practice area.

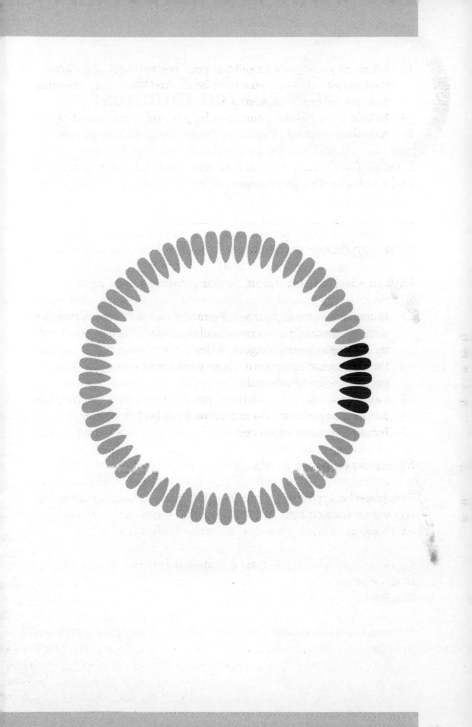

10 Only got ten minutes?

Ten minutes of regular practice promotes the flexibility of your body, as well as enhancing your balance and co-ordination.

Tadasana: spend 30 seconds grounding yourself (see the picture on page 44).

1 Stand with your feet 2–3 inches (5–10 cm) apart and your knees straight. Ensure that your body weight is distributed evenly between your two feet.
2 Lift your toes and spread them wide apart as you replace them on the ground. Close your eyes and become aware of the exchange of energy between your feet and the earth. Visualize yourself sending roots down into the earth to draw its energy up into your body.
3 Feel the energy spreading upward into your legs. Feel your shins over your heels. Make sure that your knees are straight, but not locked.
4 As the energy comes into your trunk, ensure that your hips are straight. Imagine that you are bringing your tail bone forward to meet your pelvic bone.
5 Allow your arms to relax alongside your body, with your elbows straight but soft. Be sure that your chest is lifted, your spine erect, your shoulders relaxed. Feel as though your collar bones are broadening.
6 Keep your head upright. Gaze straight ahead.

Six sun salutations

Stand in tadasana. **Inhale deeply** and prepare yourself mentally to begin.

1 **Breathe out** as you bring your palms together directly in front of your breastbone.

2 **Breathe in** as you straighten your arms and stretch them up alongside your ears. Arch your entire body backwards, keeping your knees and elbows straight.

3 **Exhale** and bend forward. Place your hands on the ground on either side of your feet. Bring your head in towards your knees. If you have difficulty reaching the ground, allow your knees to bend slightly.

4 **Inhale** as you stretch your right leg back as far as possible. Bend both knees and place the back knee on the ground. Look up, keeping your hands on the ground on either side of your left foot.

5 **Hold your breath** as you bring your left foot back in line with your right; straighten both knees so that your body is in a straight line from head to heels.

6 **Exhale** as you bend your knees and bring them directly down to the ground. Keep your hips up and drop your chest to the ground between your hands. Place your chin on the ground.

7 Without moving your hands or feet, **inhale** as you slide forward and arch into the 'cobra' pose. Keep your abdomen on the ground. Your elbows are bent slightly and in towards your sides. Your shoulders are relaxed and down, away from your ears.

8 Tuck your toes under and **breathe out** as you lift your hips high. Straighten your elbows and allow your head to hang down between your arms. Bring your chest closer to your thighs; stretch your heels to the ground.

9 **Inhale**; bend your left knee and place it on the ground. Step forward with your right foot so that your toes are in line with your fingers. Look up without lifting your hands off the ground.

10 Bring your left foot forward, next to your right; **exhale**. Lift your hips up and drop your head towards your knees. Straighten your knees as much as possible, without lifting your hands off the ground.

11 **Inhale** as you slowly straighten your body; stretch your arms forward and then up over your head. Arch back into the same position as you were in step 3.
12 **Exhale** as you lower your arms by your sides and return to tadasana.
13 In the first sun salutation, lead with your right foot. In the next one, lead with your left foot.

Repeat this sequence six times.

Shoulderstand

1 Lie on your back. Bring your legs together and raise them to a 90-degree angle.
2 Place your hands on your buttocks. Slowly walk your hands along your back, to lift the trunk of your body, until it is as straight as possible.
3 Consciously relax your calves and your feet. Hold the shoulderstand for 30 seconds, gradually increasing the time to 3 minutes.
4 Come out of the position and relax for about 30 seconds before coming into the fish pose.

(See the picture on page 97.)

The fish

1 Lie flat on your back with your legs out straight. Bring your legs and feet together.
2 Place your hands, palms downward, one under each thigh.
3 Bend your elbows, pushing them into the ground. Arch your chest upward and place the top of your head gently onto the floor. Hold the position, with your weight mainly on your

elbows. There should be very little weight on your head or neck.

4 Your chest is wide open in this position, so take advantage of this by breathing as deeply as possible.

5 To come out of the position: lift your head slightly, slide your head back and lower your back to the ground. Relax for a few moments in the corpse pose.

6 Hold the fish pose for half of the time that you held the shoulderstand. Remember to have your weight on your elbows so that there is little or no pressure on your head or neck.

(See the picture on page 78.)

The seated forward bend

1 Sit up with your legs together and straight out in front of you.

2 Inhale deeply as you stretch your arms straight up.

3 Exhale and stretch forward from your hips. Try to keep your back straight.

4 If possible, take hold of your feet or ankles. If you cannot reach them, you may want to use a strap – or hold your shins or knees.

5 Hold the position and breathe deeply. With each exhalation, feel as though some of the tension is being released from your hips – and sink forward a bit more.
Hold the position for 10 seconds, gradually increasing the time to 3 minutes.

(See the picture on page 67.)

The inclined plane

1 Sit on the ground with your legs together and straight out in front of you.

2 Place your hands flat on the ground behind your back, about 10–12 inches (approximately 30 cm) away from your buttocks. Have your fingers pointing away from your body.

3 Drop your head back and lift your hips up as high as you can. Keep your feet together and try to bring them flat onto the ground.

4 Hold the position for 10 seconds, gradually increasing the time to 1 minute.

(See the picture on page 68.)

Half spinal twist

1 Begin in a kneeling position, sitting on your heels, with your knees and feet together.

2 Drop your hips to the floor on the right side of your feet.

3 Keep your left knee (the top one) bent and bring your left leg over your right. Place your left foot flat on the floor outside your right knee.

4 Stretch your right arm up; bring it over and around your left knee.

5 Try to hold your left ankle with your right hand. If you can't reach your left ankle, hold onto your right knee (the knee on the ground). Look over your left shoulder.

6 Breathe deeply as you hold this pose. With each exhalation, feel that you are going more deeply into it.

7 Release the position and repeat on the other side.
   Hold the half spinal twist for 10–30 seconds on each side.

(See the picture on page 93.)

Preface

Is yoga for you?

Yoga is for everyone. You can practise it whatever your age, gender or physical ability. As you establish a regular routine for yourself, you will probably begin to notice how much yoga enhances your studies, increases your efficiency at work, reduces your levels of stress and frees your mind to better enjoy your spare time.

Yoga can enliven your life at any age. Nowadays there are classes for children, young adults, pregnant women, 'gentle yoga' for the over fifties and 'golden yoga' for the over seventies.

Yoga gives you the techniques to de-stress if you find yourself stressed out, and it's a gentle road to fitness if you are less active than you would like to be.

This book is meant as a general introduction to yoga. It can help you to get started – and can serve as a trusted guide as you advance. Although you may make great progress on your own, it's often advisable to practise under the supervision of a qualified teacher, who can correct and inspire you. Your teacher should understand not only the anatomy and physiology of the human body, he/she should also be teaching from direct personal experience. You might also want to consult your doctor or healthcare professional before starting your practice.

Yoga is not a theory but a practical way of life. Begin to teach yourself yoga and you will start to see the benefits for yourself.

With best wishes for your rapid advancement on the 'path',

Swami Saradananda

1

Introduction

In this chapter you will learn:
* *the philosophy of yoga*
* *the main paths to choose from*
* *the benefits of yoga.*

The philosophy and goals of yoga

Yoga is a way of seeing all life as an integrated whole. First developed in India thousands of years ago, yoga has recently travelled to the West where its ancient techniques have been warmly embraced as an effective means to counteract the stresses and strains of today's frantic pace.

Yoga aims at integrating every aspect of your body, mind and spirit. It gives you the techniques to experience the unity of all facets of your being. Yoga is both the experience of wholeness, as well as the practice by which you can attain that experience. Yoga is your progress – and the tools for overcoming whatever obstacles may temporarily stand in the way of your advancement. And yoga is an unruffled state of mind under all conditions.

Yoga is the practice of coming back to yourself and rediscovering your essential nature. It is coming to love yourself and to understand that you are not separate from the totality of the Universe. If contemporary life seems to leave you feeling isolated and disempowered, perhaps it is time for you to turn to yoga, whose very name means 'union'.

The yogic lifestyle is one of compassionate self-discipline based on the ideals of 'simple living and high thinking'. This involves a systematic training of your mind, body and emotions. With regular practice, yoga enables you to build up your inner strength and determination. It gives you the experience of absolute freedom. The goal of yoga is to enable you to liberate yourself from all suffering. Yoga is a practical system that may be used by followers of any religion or spiritual practice. It is universal in its nature – and it brings about a state of heightened awareness.

> *Evenness of mind is yoga.*
>
> *Bhagavad Gita*, chapter 2, verse 48

> *Yoga is skill in action.*
>
> *Bhagavad Gita*, chapter 2, verse 50

> *The real meaning of yoga is freedom from pain and sorrow.*
>
> *Bhagavad Gita*, chapter 6, verse 23

> *yogas cittta vritti nirodhah*
> *Yoga is the calming of the thoughts. It is the cessation of the fluctuations of consciousness.*
>
> Yoga Sutras of Patanjali, chapter 1, verse 2

Insight

The philosophy of yoga is given in a number of ancient texts of which the *Bhagavad Gita* and Patanjali's *Yoga Sutra* are probably the best known. Both were originally written in Sanskrit, but there are a number of excellent English translations available.

The main paths of yoga – which one is for you?

As we each have different personalities, our outlooks on life and preferred ways of doing things can be quite different. For this reason, different paths of yoga have evolved over the millennia.

KARMA YOGA

Karma yoga is the path of action and of service. Through acts of selflessness, you try to purify your mind and your heart. The karma yogi attempts to do all work as though it is a kind of worship. This form of yoga involves the practice of giving your hands to your work and your mind to the divine essence. If you have an outgoing nature, if you are active and energetic, you may see working in the world as your spiritual path par excellence. Examples of well-known karma yogis are Gandhi, Nelson Mandela and Martin Luther King. Volunteering to serve meals to homeless people or read to lonely elderly people are forms of selfless service. Sections of the ancient yogic text known as the *Bhagavad Gita* deal with the principles of karma yoga. Karma yoga can be summed up in the words of modern yoga master Swami Sivananda: 'Serve, love, give, purify, meditate, realize.'

BHAKTI YOGA

Bhakti yoga involves devotion and unselfish love; it is the path of the heart. Using the techniques of singing, dancing, mantra (sound energy) repetition and prayer you try to channel your emotions into feelings of devotion. When you practise bhakti, you attempt to see God everywhere and in all beings.

If you are more emotional in nature, you may be drawn to the bhakti path. Some examples of bhakti yogis are Jesus, Mother Theresa and the followers of the Hare Krishna movement. Bhakti is said to be the safest, surest, easiest and fastest path of yoga to practise at this time in history. Anyone can practise it at any time. Its ancient texts include the *Srimad Bhagavatham* and Narada's *Bhakti Sutras*.

JNANA YOGA

Jnana yoga is the philosophical approach. The Sanskrit word jnana means knowledge, insight or wisdom. Jnana yoga is considered to be the most difficult of all the paths of yoga because it requires great strength of will and intellect. It is also seen as the most direct, as there are 'no frills'. Jnana teaches that the world is unreal and illusory. Its techniques include the study of the ancient scriptures known as the Upanishads. This is done by listening to a teacher who explains the texts, reflecting on them, discussing the texts with others, asking for clarification and ultimately realizing your identity with all existence. Examples of the analytical and scholarly people who are drawn to the path of jnana yoga include J. Krishnumurthi, Ramana Maharishi, Kabalistic scholars, Jesuit priests and Benedictine monks.

RAJA YOGA

Raja yoga is the scientific, psychological approach. It is the yoga of mental self-control, often referred to as 'classical' yoga. The Sanskrit word raja translates as 'king'; this practice allows you to become the master your own mind. Patanjali lists eight limbs of yoga in his Yoga Sutras:

▶ **yama** – *your ethical relationship with society*
▶ **niyama** – *your moral relationship with yourself*
▶ **asana** – *steady posture*
▶ **pranayama** – *control of your vital energy*
▶ **pratyahara** – *the ability to draw your attention inward, away from your senses*
▶ **dharana** – *concentrating your mind*
▶ **dhyana** – *meditation*
▶ **samadhi** – *the enlightened state.*

This listing does not imply that you need to practise these limbs in order; it is not a step-by-step process. The yamas include non-violence, truthfulness, non-stealing, moderation and non-covetousness. The niyamas are purity, contentment, self-discipline, self-study (or study of the self) and surrender of the ego. They are described further in Chapter 5.

If you are introspective by nature and drawn towards meditation, you may find that raja yoga is the path for you. Many members of religious orders and spiritual communities devote themselves to meditation. However, entering an ashram or monastery is not a prerequisite for practising raja yoga.

Insight

Because it has eight limbs, Patanjali's raja yoga is sometimes referred to as 'ashtanga yoga'. In Sanskrit 'ashta' means 'eight' and 'anga' signifies 'parts'. This path of yoga is not to be confused with the 'ashtanga vinyasa yoga' that is taught by Pattabhi Jois, a modern yoga teacher.

HATHA YOGA

Hatha yoga, the most popular form of yoga in the West today, gives you the tools to strengthen and purify your physical body as the primary vehicle of your soul.

Insight

Following one path does not disallow you from including aspects of the others in your practice. As you have various facets to your personality, an integral approach, combining parts of the different paths, will probably work best.

Hatha yoga: ancient techniques for a modern lifestyle

Many people misunderstand the term 'hatha yoga' thinking it means only the physical exercises known as 'asanas'. But the goal of hatha yoga is the same as for all other forms of yoga practice: inner peace. Good health, a flexible body and decreased stress levels are all side effects of the practice of hatha yoga – very desirable and positive by-products.

Asanas and pranayama (breathing exercises) are the two main techniques of hatha yoga. They are most effective when you are also trying to live a life in keeping with the ethical and moral basis of yoga, as well as practising meditation. Hatha yoga begins with your physical body. By gaining control of the physical, you begin to control the vital energy ('prana') in your body. Hatha yoga enables you to develop the ability to make your mind calm, one pointed and in tune with the Infinite.

The techniques of hatha yoga strengthen your physical body, so that your mind is able to overcome all obstacles to inner peace and happiness. Through the practice of hatha yoga, you endeavour to purify your body, strengthen your mind and guide your emotions into positive channels. These practices give you vitality, strength and courage. They help you to shed self-destructive habits and negative ways of thinking.

Hatha yoga purifies your body and prepares it for concentration, meditation and ultimate enlightenment. In the ancient scripture known as the Hatha Yoga Pradipika, the sage Svatmarama discusses asanas as one way of beginning to bring your mind to a contemplative state. Other authoritative texts on hatha yoga include the Gheranda Samhita and Siva Samhita.

Hatha yoga has been widely studied in recent years to understand its health benefits. Many schools of hatha yoga exist, each having its own focus. For example, some emphasize alignment while others emphasize movement. Styles vary in the amount of attention they put on asana, pranayama, meditation and relaxation.

Hatha yoga allows you to open the 'chakras' (energy centres) of your body and awaken the vast potential of spiritual energy known as 'kundalini'. It offers you a way to balance the 'ha' (yang) and 'tha' (yin) energies of your body. If you are considering beginning a programme of hatha yoga in quest of better health (increased flexibility, more strength, better sleep habits, reduced pain, relaxation and stress reduction), you will not be disappointed – if you are willing to practise on a regular basis.

> **Insight**
>
> There are a number of schools and traditions of hatha yoga that are widely taught today. You may want to try several of them. For a partial listing and comparison of approaches, see pages 193–196.

EIGHT LIMBS OF HATHA YOGA

1 *Internal and external purification, including:*
   ▷ *Yamas – your ethical relationship with society*
   ▷ *Niyamas – your moral relationship with yourself*
   ▷ *Kriyas – physical cleansing exercises.*
2 *Asanas – physical exercises.*
3 *Mudras – locking the energy in, and Bandhas – sealing the energy.*
4 *Pranayama – breathing exercises; control of the vital energy known as 'prana'.*
5 *Pratyahara – stilling your mind by stopping its connection with sense perceptions.*
6 *Dharana – concentration; progression in mental control.*
7 *Chakra meditation – steadying your mind by working with the energy centres in your body.*
8 *Samadhi – the super-conscious state; the experience of Absolute Oneness.*

ENHANCING THE QUALITY OF YOUR LIFE WITH THE PRACTICE OF HATHA YOGA

Hatha yoga sees your body as a vehicle for your soul – and your body-vehicle functions best when it is kept clean, strong and healthy. Without good health, life can be unpleasant, even if you have great wealth and power. Yoga techniques are designed to enable you to maintain a state of optimum physical and mental health.

Good health may be defined as the positive state that you experience when all of the organs of your body are functioning at their maximum capacity under the intelligent control of your mind. One of the far-reaching benefits of yoga is that it helps you to develop an enhanced awareness of the general health and well-being of your body. With practice, you find yourself not only able to sense impending health problems but also able to understand what corrective actions would be most beneficial.

Benefits of hatha yoga

PHYSICAL BENEFITS

Yoga exercise first gives attention to the back, taking the view that you are as young as your spine. It provides you with a series of gentle exercises that help to increase the flexibility of the various joints of your body, especially between your vertebrae. The asanas also lengthen and release tension from your muscles; they stimulate the lubrication of your ligaments and tendons while massaging your internal organs. Both the physical practice of yoga and the meditation help you to develop enhanced muscle control and balance. The yoga practices work on the various parts of your body in an interrelated and holistic manner that brings you to a state of inner harmony.

Detoxification and improved circulation
By gently stretching your muscles and joints as well as massaging the various organs, yoga ensures that an optimum blood supply reaches all parts of your body. It also improves the functioning of your lymphatic system and flushes out toxins. Increased circulation brings added nourishment and oxygen to all the cells of your body. Evidence seems to be accumulating which suggests that the regular practice of yoga can delay the ageing process, increase your energy and give you a remarkable zeal for life.

Arthritis and general stiffness

Yoga's slow gentle exercises can provide welcome relief to painful joints. The easy stretches, especially when practised with deep breathing, tend to relieve a great deal of the muscle tension that strains your joints. Many people see yoga and meditation as the perfect anti-arthritis formula – and an overall panacea for general stiffness in the body.

Chronic illness, such as asthma or diabetes

When you suffer from a chronic illness, you tend to feel helpless and out of control. Yoga can give you the strength to look at your condition calmly and objectively. Apart from the negative consequences of your illness, there is often something positive that you can learn from the situation.

Many chronic illnesses seem to be stress related. Yoga tends to reduce levels of anxiety and stress. With the regular practice of yoga you can learn to control your own energy and direct it where it is most needed to alleviate chronic problems. You will probably find a great improvement in your sleeping patterns. Chances are that you will also find yourself with more energy and increased stamina. If you suffer from asthma and begin a yoga practice, you will probably find yourself calmer, more relaxed and less prone to shortness of breath. The breathing exercises will be of great benefit to you.

Stress

When you continually overwork your mind and body, their natural efficiency diminishes. Yoga exercises discourage violent movements and retrain your muscles to let go of tension. Breathing exercises can help to control your mood swings while developing your ability to stay calm in the most stressful situations.

Weight reduction and eating disorders

Asanas themselves do not burn large amounts of calories, but you will probably find that a regular yoga practice can be very useful in weight management. The asanas stimulate sluggish glands to increase their hormonal secretions. They work particularly on the thyroid gland, which in turn affects the metabolism of your entire body. The shoulderstand and the fish posture are especially beneficial for the thyroid gland. Yogic practices tend to reduce anxiety and lead to improved body awareness and self-confidence. This, in turn, reduces anxious and compulsive eating.

Many food obsessions and eating disorders stem from your inability to assimilate energy in healthy ways. Yoga practice enables you to efficiently work with your prana (vital energy), giving you a healthier self-image and enabling you to be more self-reliant and less 'needy' energetically.

Insight

The physical benefits are probably the ones that first inspire you to begin your yoga practice. But you may soon find yourself profiting in a number of other ways.

PSYCHOLOGICAL BENEFITS

Regular yoga practice enhances your mental clarity and calmness, increases your bodily awareness, relieves chronic stress patterns, helps you to relax your mind, centres your attention and sharpens your concentration. It removes lethargy and mental sluggishness while helping you to overcome insomnia and depression. With practice, you will develop mental poise and experience inner balance.

Many yoga practices include visualization techniques and suggest that you adopt a positive attitude towards life. While relaxing your body and calming your mind, yoga helps you to be more open to your experiences.

Concentration and efficiency

When your mind is jumpy, you waste precious mental energy. Yoga helps you to develop the ability to concentrate and tap into your vast mental resources. Along with your enhanced ability to concentrate comes increased efficiency.

Contentment

Yoga promotes contentment, the state of mental well-being that you experience when you consider the positive in all situations and all beings. It's a dynamic and constructive attitude that helps you to look at things in a new light. Contentment brings inner joy and serenity.

Contentment means being peaceful right now, even as you are busy changing your life. It enables you to live in the present moment. Don't forget about the past, but don't agonize over it. Learn from your mistakes and be peaceful in the ever-present now.

Mental steadiness

When you look at a lake, the fewer the waves and ripples the more clearly and deeply you can see into it. Yoga is the calming of your mental activities, a lessening of the inner waves and ripples of agitation. You are left with a deep sense of peace. As your thoughts subside, your mind settles into a profound silence.

General vitality

Over a period of time you will probably notice that your yoga practice has resulted in a number of positive effects on your general energy levels. Asanas (the physical exercises) and pranayama (breathing exercises) invigorate you – both mentally and physically.

SPIRITUAL BENEFITS

As your mental and physical capacities develop, your mind becomes more concentrated and more powerful. Unless there is unwavering spiritual integrity and discipline, the new-found potentials of your mind can put strong negative distractions in your path. A powerful mind, bereft of ethics and morals, often affects others in very negative ways.

Realizing that power corrupts, the ancient sages included instructions in the teachings to enable you to purify your mind and motives. These are known as the 'yamas and niyamas'. They are admonitions to practise truthfulness and non-violence;

don't steal; don't be jealous; try to control your energy; practise and purify your mind and the environment; try to be peaceful; and don't forget to study.

As yoga accelerates your spiritual progress, the need for ethical behaviour is intensified. The yamas and niyamas form the foundations of yoga. Anyone who lives with and practises these values will find their behaviour and thoughts beginning to change. The yamas and niyamas are not harsh rules, but rather a description of human potential. They offer a way to live with deeper consciousness, integrity and joy.

THE REAL GOAL OF YOGA IS HAPPINESS

You may think that your happiness comes from outside of yourself, from some object you have acquired or a goal you have achieved. But through the practice of yoga, you begin to understand that your happiness stems from the stillness that comes when your mind is free. Happiness lies within you. You may not appreciate this truism and may continue to search for happiness in the wrong places. But, eventually, after searching for many years, you will probably begin to look within yourself. Yoga can provide you with the techniques for your search.

Yoga parable: searching for happiness

A man saw his elderly neighbour in her garden, obviously distraught and looking for something. When he offered to help, the woman told him that she had dropped her glasses inside her house.
Perplexed, the man asked 'Why are you looking out here?'
'Oh, it's dark in my house,' she replied, 'so I'm looking out here in the sunlight.'

This parallels what many people do – they look for happiness in the wrong places. Yoga is a road to peace and happiness. It is a process of inner expansion and a means of complete personal transformation.

10 THINGS TO REMEMBER

1 *The ancient techniques of yoga have been warmly embraced as effective means to counteract the stresses and strains of a modern lifestyle.*

2 *The goal of yoga is inner peace and happiness.*

3 *Yoga aims at integrating every aspect of your body, mind and spirit.*

4 *Good physical and mental health tend to be positive side-effects of your yoga practice.*

5 *There are five main paths of yoga, the most popular being 'hatha yoga'.*

6 *Asanas (physical exercises) and pranayama (breathing exercises) are the two main practices of hatha yoga.*

7 *Asanas emphasize bringing flexibility to your spine.*

8 *Regular yoga practice can give you the strength to look at your situation calmly and objectively.*

9 *Yoga practice often reduces levels of anxiety and stress, as it increases your intuition and empathy. You may experience enhanced joy, patience and compassion – and an 'opening' of your heart.*

10 *You may find yourself needing less sleep when you practise yoga regularly, yet still feel more rested and energetic.*

2

Starting your practice

In this chapter you will learn:
- *how to start practising yoga*
- *when and how often to practise*
- *where and with whom to practise*
- *what you will need*
- *about safety measures.*

Starting your practice

An ounce of practice is worth a tonne of theory.

Swami Sivananda

Yoga is a disciplined adventure of self-discovery – and the best time to embark on your inner pilgrimage is right now!

The basic practices of yoga include slow gentle exercise, deep rhythmic breathing, profound relaxation, mental concentration and positive thinking with a meditative attitude. The experience can be sweet and blissful when you embark on your quest to put the theoretical knowledge of this book into practice in your daily life.

Don't wait until all the conditions in your life are perfect – things will never be perfect. All you need is a chunk of quiet time that you resolve to dedicate to your practice. Before you begin, decide how long you are going to practise. Set aside a block of time when you are not committed to doing anything else. If you have young children, nap time is perfect. Remove the pots from the stove and turn off your phone.

Before you begin, refer to the practices in Appendix 1 and choose the one that suits you. These tables are provided as guidelines and are only suggestions; you may find that you prefer to design your own routine. Some days you may feel it appropriate to skip certain asanas and add others. However, don't allow yourself to be tempted into doing only the postures that you like. You tend to enjoy what you are good at, so you might find it advisable to focus more on the poses that you don't like. These are probably the ones that are giving you trouble, but really need some extra work. One of the goals of yoga is to bring you into a state of physical and mental balance.

You may choose to practise one table until you have perfected it – or go with your feelings of the day. Some days, when you feel particularly energetic, you may choose to do a more vigorous routine. At other times, when you are tired or feeling particularly stiff, you may find it better to revert to a very basic routine. Be sure to practise several asanas from each section. Remember that stretching and counter-stretching are both very important. Don't leave out backward bends because you are feeling particularly stiff – but do leave out inversions if you are menstruating.

Insight

Don't practise immediately after you have eaten. It is best to wait at least two hours after you have had a meal. If you are planning to go to a class after work and feel very hungry, have some juice or a cup of tea to tide you over.

After you have chosen your routine, read over the descriptions of the asanas that you plan to do. After a few practice sessions you will become familiar with the poses and this will no longer be necessary.

Lie down on the ground, flat on your back, and relax before you begin your practice. This interval provides you with the space to mentally let go of whatever else you have been doing. Use this relaxation time to detach yourself from your routine thoughts and prepare yourself to practise with one-pointed enthusiasm.

When you feel centred, when your mind and body are completely relaxed, give your body a good stretch. Then sit up and begin your practice. Begin with pranayama, then go on to the asanas. Finish with a complete relaxation.

Insight

You will probably notice that you are stiffer on one side than the other. Give your tighter side extra attention, rather than giving in to your tendency to avoid working with it. Perhaps do the pose first on your stiff side then on your more flexible side – and return to the stiff side for a much-needed further stretch.

Sweating is healthy. It cleanses your pores and facilitates the detoxification of your body. The ancient yoga scriptures recommend that if you do perspire, rub the sweat into your body to create a powerful magnetic energy. Don't jump into the shower immediately after your practice; it's best to wait as least half an hour.

Yoga is much more than just a simple workout. It is a spiritual practice designed to help you to find peace in every aspect of your life.

The step-by-step instructions in this book will help you get off to a good start. But reading a book on yoga is like reading a recipe book; unless you actually cook and eat it, you can't enjoy the dinner. So, start now and practise regularly!

Insight

Yoga is about equilibrium and poise. Whenever you stretch your body in one direction, be sure to do the counter-stretch. After you stretch forward, stretch back. After stretching to the left, repeat the exercise on your right side.

When and how often

You can practise yoga at any time of day – as long as you haven't eaten for several hours. You will probably notice that your body is stiffer in the morning because you have been lying in bed all night. You may prefer to practise when you are stiffer, this will help you to work the tightness out of your body. It will ground, relax and energize your body and mind, which is a great preparation for the day ahead.

Or, you may prefer to practise in the afternoon or evening – or your circumstance in life may be such that this is the best time. Later in the day you will find that you body is much looser. You may feel that you can relax better after finishing your work for the day.

When you practise is up to you. Take some time to see when you can fit yoga into your life. Try to dedicate a specific time and develop a regular routine. When you practise for half an hour daily, you find yourself making rapid progress. If it isn't possible for you to practise daily, try to practise every second day.

Many beginners to yoga find that attending a class once or twice a week is helpful. But even if you attend class, it's still important to practise on your own on a regular basis. If you choose not to attend a class or if there's no convenient class, try to do a longer practice at least once a week.

Practise for half an hour daily; try to do an hour's practice at least once a week.

Doing a little, but practising often, is preferable to pushing yourself into doing a lot erratically or on rare occasions.

Insight

Yoga texts suggest that you don't jump into the shower immediately after you have finished your practice. Give your

(Contd)

body time to readjust. It is best to wait at least half an hour
before bathing or eating.

Where and with whom

Yoga requires absolutely no financial outlay for equipment or
classes. It's an ideal method of exercise to teach yourself. If you
move slowly, with focused awareness, there's little likelihood that
you'll hurt yourself.

All you really need is a flat, level, uncluttered surface – and the
motivation to practise.

If you choose to practise at home, practise in a well-ventilated and
comfortably heated room. Make sure that there is sufficient fresh
air, but you are not in a draught.

When the weather is warm, you might prefer to practise outside
in the fresh air. If you have a garden with a flat lawn, this is ideal.
You could practise in a park, but make sure that you are in an area
where you have a bit of seclusion and won't be disturbed.

If you are using this book, you may choose to practise alone.
However, practising with one or more friends can help you to
establish a regular routine. Make a date and set up a regular
time and place to practise – and mark it down in your diary.
The company of like-minded people can help you to keep your
intention going. You will inspire each other on the days that
you feel a bit down. The group energy will assist you in staying
focused in your practice.

Although you may wish to teach yourself yoga, even the best book
can't take the place of a qualified teacher as it isn't possible for
you to see your own mistakes. You may think that you are straight
when in fact you aren't. So, at first, you might find it helpful to
attend a few classes. Or you may choose to take a few days and go

on a yoga retreat. This can prove to be an excellent way to jump-start your yoga practice and give your life a boost.

Insight

Yoga texts strongly recommend that you seek out 'satsang'. This is the company of like-minded individuals, of people who are also interested in practising yoga. You can encourage and inspire each other.

Who can practise yoga

Anyone can benefit from a regular yoga routine, which tends to counteract many of the negative influences of modern life. Whatever your age or physical fitness, yoga can enhance your lifestyle.

If you are an adult in your middle years who works at a desk, asanas can release the physical tensions caused by hours of sitting. Breathing exercises, that increase the supply of oxygen to your brain, help to enhance your vitality and meditation improves your powers of concentration. A regular yoga practice can free you physically and mentally, while heightening your intuition and creativity.

Your children will also benefit greatly if you choose to have them practise with you. As well as being fun, yoga develops self-discipline while enhancing children's physical and mental well-being. In today's fast world, children are losing the ability to concentrate and to relax. Over-stimulated by television, video games and fast-food diets, children are rapidly being depleted of their physical as well as their creative abilities. Yoga gives children fun-filled tools to explore and strengthen their own bodies and minds.

For teenagers, yoga can help to maintain natural flexibility. If you are an adult with teenage children, encouraging them in their yoga practice gives them the inner strength to resist many of the negative influences around them – and to be able to say 'no' when it is appropriate.

There is no upper age limit on yoga practice. If you have entered your 'golden years', the slow gentle yoga exercises are perfectly suited to you. They will help you to maintain your physical mobility and may relieve many of your physical problems such as arthritis and joint stiffness. They also stimulate digestion and circulation, especially in your hands and feet. Yoga enables you to relax and promotes sound sleep.

If you are pregnant, yoga promotes good health in your body, as well as that of your unborn child. Yoga asanas can lessen the effects of such problems as increased weight, backache and depression. If you practise during your pregnancy, you will probably find that it makes your labour easier and shorter. Although many asanas have to be modified during pregnancy, their essence is perfectly suited to this time of expanded self-awareness. Pregnancy is an especially good time for meditation.

You don't need to be particularly fit to do yoga. Whatever your physical and mental ability, you can develop a yoga routine that will gradually improve with practice.

If you are a sports enthusiast, yoga can enhance and complement your abilities. Many sports build muscle strength and stamina, but only in specific areas. Yoga can help you to counteract imbalances in muscular development and enable your body and your mind to function more efficiently. Nowadays, many professional athletes practise yoga; in fact many sports teams now have their own yoga teachers.

Insight

If you are a performer, teacher, or someone who needs to make presentations at work, yoga can help you to tap into inspirational energy. Enhance your performance skills by developing a daily practice that includes the breathing exercises in particular.

What you will need

When practising outside, make sure that the ground is dry and free of rocks. If you are indoors, have a clear space that is free of furniture.

Practise on a non-slip surface. A yoga mat is a good investment, but not absolutely necessary. A folded blanket will also work, but it does tend to slip a bit.

There is no need to buy expensive yoga clothing. Wear loose comfortable clothes, preferably cotton or other natural fibre. The more your skin is free to breathe the better. Be sure that your clothing allows you the maximum range of movement – and that it doesn't bind you at the waist or crotch. Jeans are not advisable; shorts are great! Take off your belt, if you wear one.

Practise yoga in bare feet. Leave your shoes and socks outside the room or away from your practice area.

Take off your watch and jewellery. It is best to remove your glasses or contact lenses. If you have long hair, tie it back. Have a jumper handy, in case you feel cold – and a light blanket for the relaxation periods.

If you are a bit stiff you may need some cushions, a yoga strap and/or hard foam yoga blocks. Proper use of yoga props is best learned from a teacher, who can adapt the practice to your particular needs.

Safety measures

Do not practise near furniture that you might fall onto.

Move slowly. If you experience pain, stop, come out of the position, take a few breaths and then resume your practice. Pain is your body's way of warning you that something might not be good for you. However, don't let the fear of pain stop you from practising gently. Remember to always let your reach slightly exceed your grasp.

If you're pregnant, you might consider consulting a book on pregnancy yoga or working with a teacher who specializes in this field.

If you suffer from any medical condition or have any doubts as to the safety of some of the practices, it's best to consult your physician or healthcare professional. Remember that yoga is not meant to be used as a medical prescription for any condition.

10 THINGS TO REMEMBER

1 *Wait at least two hours after eating to begin your yoga practice.*

2 *Start today! Don't put off practising.*

3 *Set aside some time each day – or each week – for your yoga practice.*

4 *Lie down and relax before you begin.*

5 *Move slowly, with focused awareness.*

6 *Practise on a flat, uncluttered surface, preferable one in which there is no furniture for you to bump into.*

7 *Wear loose comfortable clothes, preferably cotton or other natural fibre.*

8 *It is best to practise in bare feet.*

9 *If you experience pain or discomfort, stop and come out of the position.*

10 *Do not use yoga as a medical prescription for any condition.*

3

The exercises – asanas

In this chapter you will learn:
- *the various yoga exercises, known as 'asanas'*
- *how to perform each of the asanas*
- *how long to hold each asana*
- *about the benefits of the asanas.*

> *When your posture (asana) is steady and comfortable, it is accompanied by the relaxation of tension. This enables you to focus on higher things.*
>
> *Yoga Sutras* of Patanjali, chapter 2, verses 46–7

Asanas are the most popular and most widely known practice of yoga in the West. If a friend tells you, 'I'm going to a yoga class', you would probably understand her to mean that she's going to do some physical exercise.

However, asanas are quite different from most other forms of physical fitness, in many ways. They do not attempt to develop your muscles through mechanical movements; instead they demand your full attention. Yoga sees your body as a vehicle for your soul in its journey towards perfection. In keeping with this vision, asanas begin their work with your physical body, but, when practised regularly, they also develop your mental capacities, broaden your consciousness and ignite your spiritual yearnings. Good health and physical fitness are an enviable by-product, but not the final objective of the practice of asanas. The real goal of yoga practice is inner peace.

Asanas emphasize slow, gentle, non-violent movements, in keeping with 'ahimsa', one of the basic tenets of yoga. This is the principle of non-violence, attempting to do no harm to any living being, in thought, word or deed. Ahimsa involves being non-competitive with others and not being too harsh or judgemental with yourself. Never force your body into any position or compel yourself to comply with anyone else's standards.

Insight

If you have the tendency to be hard on yourself and push too hard, this often carries over to your yoga practice. It is important to remember that everyone is different; try not to compare yourself with other students. Yoga is not a competitive sport.

To master the asanas, it's best to work steadily but slowly. Fast movements often result in the build-up of lactic acid in your muscles; this may leave you feeling tired and stiff. Increasing the amount of oxygen you bring into your cells can neutralize this lactic acid. This is one of the reasons that asanas are usually accompanied by an emphasis on deep breathing. Each asana is a position that puts pressure on a certain point or points, much as acupuncture and shiatsu do. As you hold the pose, you breathe deeply. Rather than thinking about something else, you actually focus on the tension and consciously 'breathe' it out of your body. You begin to develop your abilities to control your own body by using your mind.

Rather than burning up energy, as most forms of physical exercise do, asanas tend to leave you feeling invigorated and more energetic than when you began. This is because they enable you to let go of tension that you have been holding in your muscles. With practice, asanas assist you in releasing your energetic blockages. The energy that was stagnating becomes usable; it begins to circulate throughout your body and you feel invigorated.

Asanas work on every aspect of your physical being, not just your muscles and joints. They massage your internal organs, stimulate circulation and enhance respiration. They also make your mind steady, concentrated and ready for meditation.

A better translation for the word 'asanas' would be pose, position or seat. The term implies much more than physical exercise. Its roots are connected to the idea of being fully present in the moment and being firmly grounded in your body.

There are two directions for you to use when approaching the asanas. If you take yoga classes, you will notice that some schools work from the top down; other traditions start from the bottom and work up. If you think of asanas as purely physical exercises, neither method seems to make any difference. But, when you understand the benefits of asanas in relation to your subtle energies, you see that where you start and in which direction you work is very important.

When you practise standing poses first, you begin at the bottom, with the lowest chakras (page 176). In this approach, you attempt to ground yourself and then work upwards. You finish your session with inverted positions, such as the shoulderstand and headstand, where the focus is on the higher energy centres. Working this way leaves you more ready to do abstract work – or to sit for meditation.

Alternatively, you can start with the inverted poses and work downward, finishing with standing positions. This leaves you feeling grounded and ready to actively work in the world. The choice of direction is up to you. We have included samples of each approach in the practices in Appendix 1. You may want to use them on different days, depending on what you are hoping to achieve in your practice.

General guidelines for your asana practice
▶ *Begin by relaxing your muscles – then warming them up.*
▶ *Before you attempt an asana, make sure that you understand the theory of how it is performed.*
▶ *Stretch your body in one direction, and then stretch it the opposite way.*

- ▶ *Don't hold back or try to save your energies. Be generous with yourself. Remember that the more energy you put into your practice, the more you get back.*
- ▶ *Work from where you are, with what you have. Your experiences and previous training make you distinct from everyone else. Try not to compare yourself with others. Yoga is non-competitive.*
- ▶ *Come into each position slowly and gradually. Do not jump into the poses nor try to force yourself into them. Do not move carelessly; try to consciously connect with each movement.*
- ▶ *At first, practise each asana for a shorter period; gradually increase the amount of time that you hold it.*
- ▶ *Let your reach slightly exceed your grasp, but stop before you experience pain.*
- ▶ *Breathe deeply as you hold each pose.*
- ▶ *Use your breath to relax, and try to relax into every pose.*
- ▶ *As you hold the position, check your body mentally. If you find tension anywhere in your body, try to consciously 'breathe' it out.*
- ▶ *End your session with a relaxation that encourages your energies to flow unimpeded throughout your entire body.*
- ▶ *Enjoy your practice!*

Warming up

THE SUN AND THE MOON

When beginning to do the 'asanas', the physical exercises, you will probably find it helpful to remember that hatha yoga is a unifying practice. The word 'yoga' means union or self-discipline. Hatha yoga is a symbolic union of sun and moon – the opposing forces in nature. It is an integration of the male and female principles, which are present within each of us. In the Chinese context, this is expressed as the yin and yang; in the Indian tradition it's referred to as Siva and Shakti. The practice of yoga asanas helps you to achieve a unity of body and mind, a great aid in today's fragmented world.

If you are stiff, especially if you are practising in the early morning, you may want to give your body a good shake before beginning. Let your fingers go limp and shake them from the wrists. Then shake your arms and legs. Roll your shoulders, circling forward and then back.

NECK STRETCHES

These may be done when you are sitting or standing.

1 *Forward and back. Drop your head down towards your chest, so that your chin touches (or almost touches) your breast bone. Then bring your head back as far as you can, lifting your chin and visualizing the back of your head touching your spine. Repeat these movements 3–4 times in each direction, and then return your head to its upright position.*
2 *Side to side. Stretch your head straight down to the left; imagine that you are trying to get your left ear to touch your left shoulder. Don't allow your neck to twist or your shoulders to rise. Then stretch your head to the right. Repeat these movements 3–4 times in each direction, and then return your head to its upright position.*
3 *Twist your head from side to side. Without moving your shoulders, turn your head to the right, as though you are trying to see behind your back. Then turn to the left. Repeat these movements 3–4 times in each direction; return your head to its upright position.*

Now you are ready to begin your asana practice.

Insight

There are many different warm-up 'salutations'. The ones given here are among the simplest and most popular. However, be aware that different schools of yoga teach different routines.

SUN SALUTATION (FIGURE 3.1)

The traditional wisdom that 'you are as young as your spine' defines the primary benefit of this excellent 12-part warm-up exercise. The sun salutation sequence stretches your spine forward and back, while promoting flexibility in your other limbs as well. Each position is connected with your breathing and helps you to regulate your breath for the rest of the day.

If you are a complete beginner and find that there are too many things to remember, try to learn the body positions first. Once you're familiar with the sequence, try to co-ordinate your movements with your breath in order to obtain the maximum benefit. Enjoy the flowing dance-like movements!

The sun salutation is a powerful aid that helps you to focus your mind and prepare it for your asana session, as well as for your day ahead. It's traditionally done first thing in the morning, facing the sun (if possible) or facing eastward.

When to do: at the beginning of your asana practice. On the days that you're particularly short of time, try to at least do six sun salutations, even if you don't have time to practise anything else.

Benefits of the sun salutation
- ▶ *The sun salutation is an excellent warm-up exercise that gives your body an all-over initial stretch. It prepares you mentally and physically for your asana practice.*
- ▶ *The various spinal positions give a full range of vertebral movement to your spine.*
- ▶ *It regulates your breathing and helps you to focus your mind.*
- ▶ *It recharges the chakra (energy centre) at your solar plexus region.*
- ▶ *The slow, rhythmic breathing stimulates your cardiovascular system.*
- ▶ *Beginners, elderly and those with stiff joints will notice a rapid increase in general flexibility with regular practice of the sun salutation.*

How to do the sun salutation
Stand erect in tadasana (see page 44). Have your feet together and your arms relaxed by the side of your body. Inhale deeply and prepare yourself mentally to begin.

1 Breathe out as you bring your palms together directly in front of
   your breastbone in the classical 'namaskar', or prayer position.
   This movement helps to you to centre both your body and your
   mind (Figure 3.1a). Note: In 'namaskar' your hands are in front
   of your heart centre; this is the energetic centre of your body.

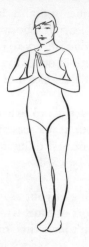

Figure 3.1a.

2 Breathe in as you straighten your elbows and stretch your
   arms straight up alongside your ears. Your hands are high
   up over your head with your palms facing each other.
   Simultaneously, arch your entire body backwards, keeping
   your knees and elbows straight. This is a complete stretch for
   your body – from fingers to heels (Figure 3.1b).

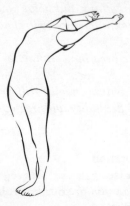

Figure 3.1b.

3 *Exhale and bend forward. Place your hands on the ground on either side of your feet. Bring your head in towards your knees. If you are unable to reach the ground with your knees straight, allow your knees to bend, but only as much as is necessary (Figure 3.1c).*

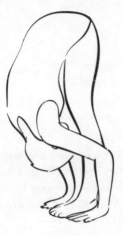

Figure 3.1c.

4 *Inhale as you stretch your right leg back as far as possible. Bend both knees and place the back knee on the ground. Look up, keeping your hands on the ground on either side of your left foot (Figure 3.1d).*

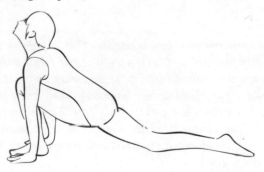

Figure 3.1d.

5 *Hold your breath as you bring your left foot back in line with your right; straighten both knees. Your body is now in a*

'push-up' position, with your back and legs forming a straight line from the head to the heels (Figure 3.1e).

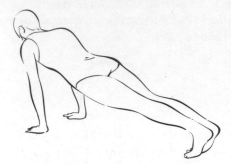

Figure 3.1e.

6 Exhale as you bend your knees and bring them directly downwards until they are on the ground. Keep your hips up and drop your chest to the ground between your hands. Place your chin (or your forehead, if you are more flexible) on the ground (Figure 3.1f).

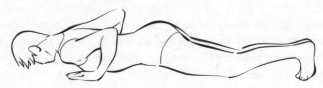

Figure 3.1f.

7 Without moving your hands or your feet, inhale as you slide your body forward and arch up with your head and chest. This is known as the 'cobra' pose and may be practised by itself as a separate asana (see page 80). Your body is on the ground from the waist downward. Your hands are flat on the ground. Your elbows are bent slightly and in towards your sides. Your shoulders are relaxed and down, away from your ears (Figure 3.1g).

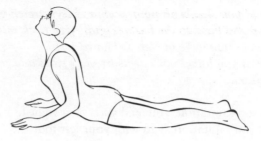

Figure 3.1g.

8 *Tuck your toes under and breathe out as you lift your hips as high as possible. Do not move your hands or feet. Straighten your elbows and allow your head to hang down between your arms. Bring your chest closer to your thighs, as you stretch your heels to the ground. This position, popularly known as 'downward dog' (page 42), may be practised on its own or as part of the sun salutation (Figure 3.1h).*

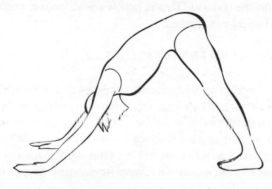

Figure 3.1h.

9 *Inhale and bend your left knee down to the ground. Almost simultaneously, step forward with your right foot. Make sure that the toes of your right foot are in line with the tips of your fingers. Look up without lifting your hands off the ground (Figure 3.1d).*

10 *Bring your left foot forward, next to your right; exhale. Lift your hips up and drop your head down towards your knees. Straighten your knees as much as possible, without lifting your hands off the ground (Figure 3.1c).*

11 *Inhale as you slowly straighten your body; stretch your arms forward and then up over your head. Arch back into the same position as you were in step 2 (Figure 3.1b).*

12 *Exhale as you lower your arms by your sides and return to tadasana.*

In this first sun salutation, you lead with your right foot. When you do the next sun salutation, lead with your left foot.

How many/how long: begin by doing six sun salutations daily. Try to gradually increase it to 12 rounds.

Remember: to do an even number of rounds of the sun salutation to ensure equal stretching on both sides.

Caution: if you are pregnant, do a modified sun salutation in which you don't lift your arms over your head nor rest your abdomen (stomach) on the ground. This is best learned from a teacher who specializes in pregnancy yoga.

MOON SALUTATION (FIGURE 3.2)

To balance the activating dynamic energy of the sun, the moon salutation cultivates a calming, rejuvenating quality which is usually associated with the divine feminine. This 16-part warm-up exercise is best done as part of an afternoon/evening practice. While the sun salutation works vertically, stretching your spine forward and back, the moon salutation works on a more horizontal, deeper plane.

When to do: at the start of your asana practice.

Benefits of the moon salutation
▶ *The flowing movements of the moon salutation calm and cool your nervous system.*
▶ *It brings balance into your life on a variety of levels: physical, psychological and spiritual.*
▶ *It's particularly beneficial for women to practise during menstruation, pregnancy and menopause.*

- ▶ *Its earthy squats help you to feel more grounded.*
- ▶ *All parts of your body, including some that you never knew you had, are stretched and invigorated.*

How to do the moon salutation

Stand erect with your feet 5–10 cm apart, making sure that your weight is evenly distributed. Relax your arms by the side of your body. Take a few deep breaths as you prepare yourself mentally to begin.

1 *Inhale as you raise your arms straight out to the sides and then over your head in a lateral, circular motion. When your palms meet, interlock your fingers, and then release your index fingers so that they are pointing upward. Make sure to keep your elbows straight; try to have your arms behind your ears as much as possible. Stretch your entire body upwards, keeping your chin up, away from your chest (Figure 3.2a).*

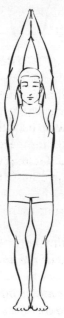

Figure 3.2a Moon salutation.

2 *Half moon to the right: look straight ahead as you stretch
your entire body upward. Keeping this stretch, exhale as you
bend towards the right. Push your left hip to the left; do not
allow your body to twist. Check yourself to make sure that
your weight is distributed equally on both feet – and your
chin is away from your chest. Inhale as you return to centre
(Figure 3.2b).*

   *Half moon to the left: exhale as you bend to the left. Inhale as
you come back to centre.*

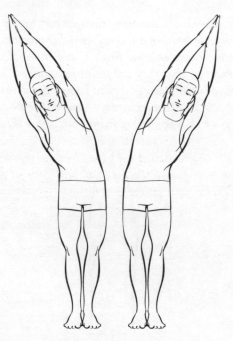

Figure 3.2b.

3 *Kali squat: stepping with your right foot, come into a wide
stance. Have your feet wider than your hips, at least 60 cm
apart. Rotate your toes out to a 45-degree angle. Bend your
knees and sit down as much as possible, keeping your back
straight. Do not allow your knees to drop inward, keep them
so that they are over your feet. Tuck your tail bone under.
Simultaneously, unclasp your hands, bend your elbows and
lower your arms. Have your elbows in line with your shoulders*

*(not in front or behind). Your fingers are still pointing upward;
your palms are facing inwards, framing your face (Figure 3.2c).*

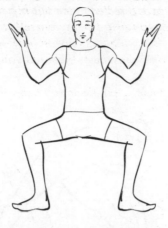

Figure 3.2c.

4 *Starfish: straighten your knees and straighten your feet – have
your toes facing forward and your feet parallel. Straighten
your elbows and stretch your arms straight out from your
shoulders with your palms downwards (Figure 3.2d).*

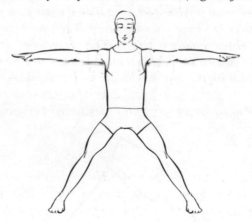

Figure 3.2d.

5 *Triangle: turn your right foot and thigh 90 degrees to the right;
turn your left foot in slightly. With your arms straight out from
your shoulders, stretch your arms and upper body to the right*

*as much as possible. Then lower your right hand and catch
hold of your right ankle or shin. Keep your arms in a straight
line, with your gaze directed at the upper hand (Figure 3.2e).*

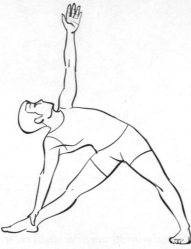

Figure 3.2e.

6 *Runner's stretch: turn to face your right. Rotate your back
   foot until both of your feet are parallel, with your right foot
   in front. Try to have your hips even. Turn your entire body
   to the right and place both hands on the ground (if possible)
   on either side of your right foot. If you are unable to place
   your hands on the ground, hold your right ankle or shin with
   both hands. Bring your head down towards your right shin.
   Remember to keep both your knees straight (Figure 3.2f).*

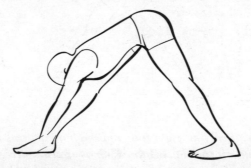

Figure 3.2f.

7 *Right lunge: bend both knees. Drop your back (left) knee to the ground and bring both of your hands to the floor on either side of your front (right) foot. Look up (Figure 3.2g).*

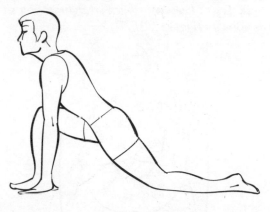

Figure 3.2g.

8 *Right squat: bring both of your hands in front of your right foot as you pivot to face forward. Try to keep your right knee directly over the foot. Rotate your left foot until it's resting on the heel with your toes pointing straight upwards (Figure 3.2h).*

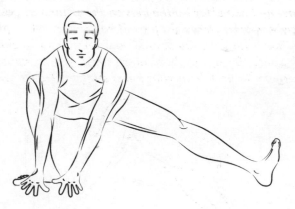

Figure 3.2h.

9 *Central, deep squat: walk your hands to the centre, in front of your body. Bring both feet flat on the ground and turn your*

toes out to a 45-degree angle (as in the kali squat). Bend your elbows and use them to push your knees outwards. Bring the palms of your hands together in 'prayer' position in front of your chest. Try to keep your back straight as you sit down as much as you can (Figure 3.2i).

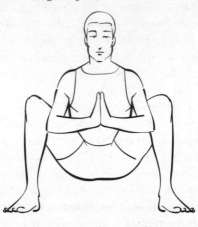

Figure 3.2i.

10   Left squat: replace your hands on the floor and walk them to the left until they are in front of your left foot. Try to have your left knee directly over the foot. Rotate your right foot until it is resting on the heel and your toes are pointing straight upwards (Figure 3.2j).

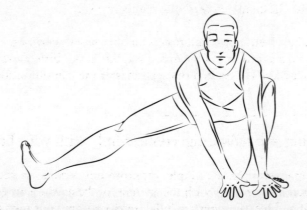

Figure 3.2j.

11   *Left lunge: pivot to face your left foot. Drop your back (right) knee to the ground and bring both hands to the floor on either side of your front (left) foot (see Figure 3.2g).*

12   *Runners stretch: straighten both knees. Make sure that your hips are straight and your feet are parallel, with your left foot in front. Both hands remain on the ground (if possible) on either side of your left foot. If you are unable to keep your hands on the ground, hold your left ankle or shin with both hands. Bring your head down towards your left shin (see Figure 3.2f).*

13   *Triangle: bring your right arm up, returning to the triangle position (see Figure 3.2e).*

14   *Starfish: inhale as you use your right arm to straighten up. Have your toes pointing forward with your feet parallel. Both arms are stretching straight out from your shoulders palms downwards (see Figure 3.2d).*

15   *Kali squat: turn your toes out to a 45-degree angle. Bend your knees, bend your elbows and sit down as much as possible. Keep your chest up, your back straight and your tail bone tucked under (see Figure 3.2c).*

16   *Half moon: bring your hands together and release the index fingers. Step your feet almost together. Stretch to your right and then to the left. Be sure to keep your weight evenly balanced on both feet as you do this (see Figure 3.2b).*

How many/how long: do at least two moon salutations. Start the first moon salutation by bending to the right and the second to your left. Gradually increase the number to six.

Remember: the moon salutation is an alternative warm-up exercise to the sun salutation. As the moon salutation is a little more complicated, it's suggested that you master the sun salutation first.

Standing and balancing: connect fully with your body

Standing up straight is a simple, yet profound, action. As you stand, you connect your body with the energies of the earth. You ground yourself and feel that you are fully present within your own body.

Include at least 2–3 of the following standing poses in your yoga session. Practise them together, one after the other, in a standing series.

DOWNWARD-FACING DOG (FIGURE 3.3)

This is one of simplest of the asanas, yet a very powerful pose. Some people consider this position to be an introversion, as your head is downward.

When to do: this is best done at the beginning of your asana practice – or just after the warming-up exercises. Downward-facing dog is also a valuable transition asana, helping you to move smoothly from one pose to another.

Benefits of the downward-facing dog pose
- ▸ *Your body is grounded and prepared for asana practice.*
- ▸ *Hamstrings and all the muscles of the back of your legs are stretched.*
- ▸ *There is no pressure on your breathing mechanism; the position encourages you to breathe deeply and fully.*
- ▸ *Arms and shoulders are strengthened.*
- ▸ *Shoulder and upper back flexibility are encouraged.*

How to do the downward-facing dog pose

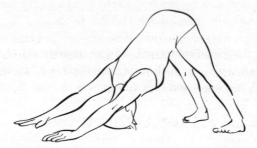

Figure 3.3 Downward-facing dog.

1 *Come onto your hands and knees; have your hands directly under your shoulders with your elbows straight. Have your legs apart with your knees directly beneath your hips.*

2 *Tuck your toes under and slowly straighten your knees.*
   Lift your hips and bring your chest as close to your thighs
   as possible.
3 *Try to bring your heels as close to the ground as possible.*
   If your heels come down easily, you may find it helpful to step
   back a bit more to get the full benefit of the pose. If your heels
   are nowhere near the floor, don't worry about it. They'll get
   there with practice.
4 *Breathe deeply and hold the pose (Figure 3.3). When you are*
   ready to come out of it, bend your knees and bring them down
   to the ground.

How many/how long: hold downward-facing dog for at least
30 seconds. Gradually increase the time to 3 minutes. If you find
that you are getting tired, come out of the pose, rest for about
10 seconds in child's pose (see page 112) and then come back into
downward-facing dog.

Remember: keep your hands flat on the ground. Push both
hands and feet down so that your weight is evenly distributed on
all four.

Caution: if you are a beginner or if you are menstruating, you may
want to practise downward-facing dog in place of inverted poses
(pages 96–108).

Insight

You can practise the downward-facing dog in place of
inverted poses, such as headstand and shoulderstand, when
you are menstruating. Although your head is down in the
pose, your body is not totally inverted.

TADASANA – STEADY AS THE MOUNTAIN
(FIGURE 3.4)

Tadasana is the perfect foundation on which you can begin to
build a regular asana practice. As you hold the pose, your feet are
grounding you as your body stretches up towards the sky.

When to do: at the beginning of your asana practice; also between asanas.

Benefits of tadasana, the mountain pose
- *Physical balance and mental poise are enhanced.*
- *You become aware of your posture and the alignment of your spine.*
- *You experience fully your connection with the earth and its energies.*

How to do tadasana pose

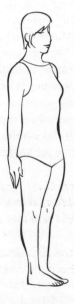

Figure 3.4 Tadasana.

1 *Stand firmly with your feet 2–3 inches (5–10 cm) apart and your knees straight. Be aware of the four corners of each foot: the ball under your big toe, the outer edge of the front of your foot, your inner heel and your outer heel. Imagine that you are pushing all of these corners into the ground. Feel your body weight spread evenly between your feet.*

2 *Without lifting your foot itself, lift your toes and spread them wide apart. Replace your toes on the ground. Close your eyes*

and become aware of the exchange of energy between your feet and the earth. You may find it helpful to visualize yourself sending roots down into the earth to draw its energy up into your body.

3 *Close your eyes and stand for a moment to experience your balance. Shift slightly from one foot to the other; make sure that your weight is evenly distributed between your two feet. Then gently rock forward and back until you find your point of balance. Allow your weight to come to the inside of each foot and then the outside – make sure that you are evenly balanced within each foot as well.*

4 *Feel the energy spreading upward into your legs. Feel your shins over your heels. Make sure that your knees are straight, but not locked.*

5 *As the energy comes into your trunk, ensure that your hips are straight. Imagine that you are bringing your tail bone forward to meet your pelvic bone.*

6 *Allow your arms to relax alongside your body, with your elbows straight but soft. Be sure that your chest is lifted, your spine erect, your shoulders relaxed. Feel as though your collar bones are broadening.*

7 *Have your head upright. Gaze straight ahead (Figure 3.4). Breathe deeply and hold tadasana, constantly re-checking your body to make sure that it remains straight.*

How many/how long: practise tadasana for as long as you like. It's an asana in itself and also the starting point for many of the other poses.

Remember: to keep your weight evenly distributed between your feet.

STANDING FORWARD BEND (FIGURE 3.5)

From the upwardly mobile tadasana, fold your body in half and bring your head close to the earth.

When to do: at the beginning of your standing asanas, just after tadasana.

Benefits of the standing forward bend

▶ *Spinal flexibility.*
▶ *Stretches hamstrings and the other muscles in the backs of your legs.*
▶ *This is a full forward bend, involving your entire body.*
▶ *Enhances your concentration.*
▶ *Brings you humility and a more introverted attitude.*

How to do standing forward bend

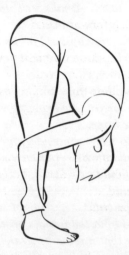

Figure 3.5 Standing forward bend.

1 *Stand erect in tadasana, with your feet 2–3 inches (5–10 cm) apart.*
2 *Inhale as you lift your arms up alongside your ears. Have your elbows straight and your arms straight up over your head.*
3 *Exhale as you bend forward and down as far as possible. Keep your knees straight.*
4 *If possible, catch hold of your ankles. If you can't reach your ankles, hold the backs of your shins or knees.*
5 *Breathe as you remain in the position, with your weight on the balls of your feet. Lift your hips as high as possible (Figure 3.5).*

How many/how long: hold for 10 seconds, gradually increasing to 1 minute.

Remember: to keep your weight evenly distributed between your feet; do not allow your knees to bend.

Caution: do not attempt the standing forward bend if you have a cold or if your nose is blocked for any reason. If you are pregnant, practise this pose with your legs wider apart.

Variations of the standing forward bend
Variation 1
For beginners, a simple variation to the forward bend is to simply hang forward and clasp each elbow with the opposite hand. Keep your knees straight and allow the weight of your head to gradually enhance your stretch.

Variation 2
An advanced variation is to place your hands on the ground on either side of your feet. Try to gradually bring your hands as flat on the ground as possible and attempt to have the upper half of your body resting against your legs.

Variation 3
A more advanced pose is to lift the fronts of your feet as you bend forward. Stand on your heels and slide your hands under the respective soles of your feet, with your palms upwards. Bring your head in towards your shins as you shift your weight forward as much as possible. Keep your knees straight and your hips high.

Variation 4
An even more advanced position is to reach back behind your calves and clasp each of your elbows with the opposite hand. Bring your head and upper body in towards your shins.

Caution: do not attempt advanced variations until you have mastered the simple pose – and don't do them if you're pregnant.

CHAIR (FIGURE 3.6)

This is an excellent asana for exploring the movement potential of
your lower spine and pelvic region.

When to do: after standing forward bend.

Benefits of the chair pose
▶ *Stretches your hamstrings.*
▶ *Brings physical balance and mental concentration.*

How to do the chair pose

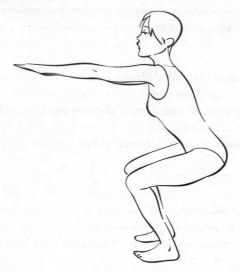

Figure 3.6 The chair.

1 *Stand in tadasana. Bring your feet approximately 15 cm apart but keep them parallel to each other. Look at a point straight in front of you.*
2 *Bring your arms straight out in front of you. Have them at shoulder level, parallel to the floor with your palms facing downward.*
3 *Keeping your heels on the ground as much as possible, bend your knees and feel as though you are about to sit down on an invisible chair.*
4 *Take a few breaths; hold the position for a moment.*
5 *Lean back a bit and try to sit down a bit more. Try to keep your chest up as much as possible. Tuck your tail bone in (Figure 3.6).*
6 *Repeat steps 4 and 5 several times.*

How many/how long: try to hold the chair pose for at least 10 seconds, then come out of it and relax for a moment. Repeat this 2–5 times.

Remember: there are many variations to the chair pose. If your shoulders and upper back are more flexible, you may try doing the chair pose with your arms straight up and your palms facing each other.

TRIANGLE (FIGURE 3.7)

This is a standing pose that gives a lateral stretch.

When to do: as part of your standing series.

Benefits of the triangle pose
▶ *Enables your spine and back muscles to stretch laterally.*
▶ *Brings hip flexibility.*
▶ *Improves circulation.*
▶ *Regular practice helps you to maintain a youthful gait.*
▶ *Improves concentration.*

How to do the triangle pose

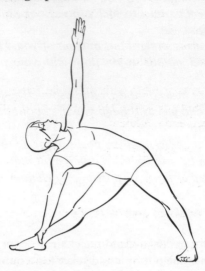

Figure 3.7 The triangle.

1 *Step your feet wide apart. Make sure that they are wider than your shoulders.*
2 *Raise your arms straight out to the sides. Have them at shoulder level, parallel to the ground with your palms facing downwards.*
3 *Turn your right foot out to a 90-degree angle and rotate your left foot inwards to a 45-degree angle.*
4 *Keeping your arms up, lengthen your rib cage to your right. Extend your right arm out over your right leg, without letting your body twist. Move to your right as much as possible.*
5 *Reach down with your right hand to hold your right ankle. If you can't reach your ankle, hold your shin or thigh. Think of your arms, shoulders and collar bones as comprising a single unit with no joints. As your right arm goes down, your left arm stretches straight up.*
6 *Lift your left hip. Stretch your left arm up towards the ceiling; look up at your left hand (Figure 3.7).*
7 *Breathe deeply; hold the pose. Release it and repeat the triangle on the other side.*

How many/how long: 10 seconds on each side, gradually increasing the time to 30 seconds. You may repeat the pose 2–3 times on each side.

Remember: to not twist your body.

Caution: if you have trouble with this pose, keep your left hand on your left hip as you attempt it. Don't raise your left arm until you feel fully balanced and confident.

ROTATED TRIANGLE (FIGURE 3.8)

A challenging, yet fun variation of the basic pose.

When to do: an optional pose after the triangle.

Benefits of the rotated triangle pose
- ▶ *Tones your spinal nerves and abdominal organs.*
- ▶ *Increases peristalsis which improves digestion. Rotating to your left will gently massage your ascending colon.*
- ▶ *Your spine is stretched laterally.*
- ▶ *Stimulates your energy in the solar plexus region.*

How to do the rotated triangle pose

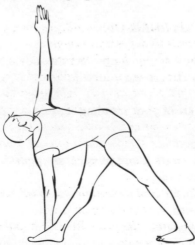

Figure 3.8 Rotated triangle.

1 Stand with your feet slightly more than shoulder-width apart. Have your feet parallel with your toes facing straight ahead.
2 Extend your arms straight out to the sides at shoulder height, with your elbows straight.
3 Twist from your waist, rotating your upper body to face the right. Place your left hand on the floor outside your right foot. (Use a block if you are unable to place your hand on the ground.)
4 Stretch your right arm straight up and look up at your right hand. The fingers of your right hand should be pointing up towards the ceiling (Figure 3.8).
5 Hold the pose; release; repeat on the other side.

How many/how long: begin by holding each side for at least 10 seconds, gradually increasing the time until you are holding for 30 seconds.

Remember: think of your arms, shoulders and collar bones as comprising a single unit with no joints.

Caution: practise the triangle pose for a while before attempting this variation.

WARRIOR 1 (FIGURE 3.9)

This intense classical standing pose does wonders for your general posture and ability to ground yourself.

When to do: as part of your standing series.

Benefits of warrior 1
▶ *Mental concentration and physical strength.*
▶ *Legs are stretched.*
▶ *Chest is expanded and breathing enhanced.*
▶ *Hips are opened.*
▶ *Thighs are strengthened.*
▶ *You establish a strong, rooted foundation for your practice – and for your life.*

How to do warrior 1

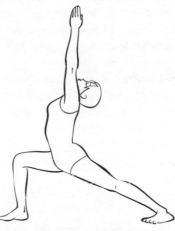

Figure 3.9 Warrior 1.

1 *Stand in tadasana, but with your feet 5–10 cm apart. Place your hands on your hips and ensure that your hips do not twist as you do the following.*
2 *Step forward with your right foot. Turn your left foot in slightly. Step forward again with your right foot as you bend your right knee. Bring your feet at least 1 metre apart and your right thigh parallel to the ground. The more you can step apart, the easier this is to do.*
3 *Ensure that your front knee is directly over your front foot – don't let your knee push forward. Keep your back knee straight. Bring your arms straight up over your head, with the palms facing each other. Don't lean forward; keep your trunk upright and your weight equally distributed on both feet. Breathe deeply as you hold the position (Figure 3.9).*
4 *Come back to tadasana and repeat the pose in the opposite direction.*

How many/how long: try to hold the pose for 10 seconds on each side, gradually increase it to 1 minute. Repeat on other side.

Remember: keep your hips even, with both hips facing in the same direction as your feet.

Caution: be careful with this pose if you have knee problems.

WARRIOR 2 (FIGURE 3.10)

This is an excellent pose in which to explore the balance and relationship between your legs.

When to do: after warrior 1.

Benefits of warrior 2
▸ *Same as warrior 1, but more so!*

How to do warrior 2

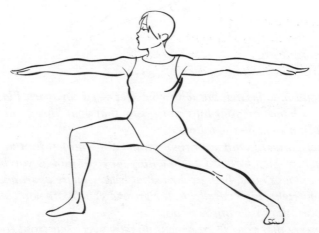

Figure 3.10 Warrior 2.

1 *Come into warrior 1.*
2 *Bring your arms down to shoulder level, parallel to the ground with your palms facing downwards.*
3 *Thinking of your arms, shoulders and collar bones as a single unit, twist your upper body to your left. Twist until your arms are directly over your legs. Gaze at your right hand and breathe deeply as you hold the position (Figure 3.10).*

How many/how long: try to hold for 10 seconds on each side, gradually increasing to 1 minute. Repeat on the other side.

Remember: don't lean forward; keep your trunk upright and your weight equal on both feet.

Caution: be careful with this pose if you have knee problems.

NATARAJA – THE ETERNAL DANCER (FIGURE 3.11)

Practising this beautiful asana brings you great inner poise in addition to its other mental and physical benefits.

When to do: as part of your standing poses.

Benefits of nataraja
▶ *Your body becomes light and graceful.*
▶ *Your hip flexors open and strengthen.*
▶ *Your mind and body develop balance.*

How to do nataraja

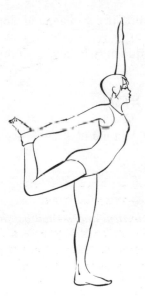

Figure 3.11 Nataraja.

1 *Stand in tadasana and bend your right knee so that your right foot comes up towards your right buttock.*
2 *Reach down with your right arm and take hold of your right ankle.*
3 *Stretch your left arm straight up, alongside your left ear.*
4 *Imagine that your body is one solid piece from your bent knee up to your upper fingers. Fix your gaze on a point about 2 metres in front of your toes.*
5 *Gradually begin to lift your bent knee. As you do this, your entire body will tilt forward in one piece.*
6 *Keep lifting the bent knee until your body is parallel with the ground. Balance in this position, breathing gently (Figure 3.11).*
7 *Release the pose and repeat on the other side.*

How many/how long: try to hold the position for 10 seconds on each side, gradually increasing to 30 seconds.

Remember: to keep your arm straight and alongside your ear.

Caution: if you have difficulty balancing in this pose, practise in front of a wall.

TREE (FIGURE 3.12)

Start with a firm foundation and allow yourself to 'grow' upwards.

When to do: anytime!

Benefit of the tree pose
▶ *Enhances your physical and mental balance.*

How to do the tree pose

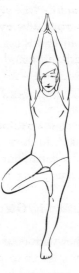

Figure 3.12 The tree.

1 *Stand in tadasana. Bend your right knee and place the sole of your right foot flat against your inner left thigh.*
2 *Keep your left knee straight and your left leg steady.*
3 *Bring your palms together at your chest. Slowly straighten your elbows and extend your arms straight up over your head. Make sure that your palms stay together.*
4 *Look straight ahead and hold the position, balancing on your left foot. As you hold the position, feel as though your right foot is sending roots down into the ground. Be aware of the gravity of the earth. Rather than resisting the downward pull, feel as though it is assisting you in standing more firmly (Figure 3.12).*
5 *Lower your right foot and your arms. Return to tadasana and repeat the pose on the other side.*

How many/how long: start by holding the tree pose for 10 seconds on each side. Gradually build up to 1 minute.

Remember: to keep your balance by fixing your gaze on a point on the ground approximately 1 metre in front of your feet.

Caution: if you have difficulty balancing, stand with your left side about 15 cm away from a wall. Place your left hand on the wall and come into the tree position. When you feel ready, release from the wall and bring your hands together over your head. When you have finished on this side, turn and repeat the pose on the other side.

Insight

There is a Chinese proverb that 'to be healthy you need both the earth and the sky'. In the tree pose, your feet are connecting firmly with the earth, but your energy is lifting you up towards the heavens.

KNEELING CRESCENT MOON (FIGURE 3.13)

This pose may be done either with your arms over your head or at shoulder level.

When to do: as part of your standing or backward bending series.

Benefits of kneeling crescent moon
- ▶ *Hips are opened.*
- ▶ *Balance and concentration are improved.*
- ▶ *Chest is expanded and breathing enhanced.*

How to do kneeling crescent moon

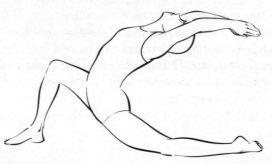

Figure 3.13 Kneeling crescent moon.

1 *Stand on your knees.*
2 *Place your right foot flat on the floor in front of you. Ensure that your foot is directly under your knee and your thigh parallel to the ground.*
3 *Bring your palms together at the chest in prayer pose, also known as the 'namaskar' position.*
4 *Keeping your palms together and your elbows straight, stretch your arms up. Arch back as far as possible. Make sure that the front foot stays flat on the floor. Feel as though you are lifting from the front thigh (Figure 3.13).*

How many/how long: hold the pose for about 10–30 seconds, then repeat it on the other side.

Remember: to keep your knee directly over your foot; do not permit your knee to push forward.

Caution: if you are pregnant, this pose is best practised with your arms straight out from your shoulders and parallel to the ground.

CROW (FIGURE 3.14)

Imagine your hands as crow's feet.

When to do: anytime.

Benefits of the crow pose
▶ *Helps you to develop mental and physical balance.*
▶ *Strengthens your forearms and wrists.*
▶ *Brings flexibility to your wrists and fingers. The crow is a powerful pose to counteract many of the negative effects of working at a computer.*

How to do the crow pose

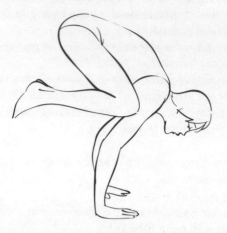

Figure 3.14 The crow.

1 *Come into a squatting position, with your knees wide apart.*
2 *Spread your fingers wide. Place your palms flat on the ground with your hands rotated inward slightly and your elbows bent outward. If you are more advanced and/or stronger you may attempt the crow with your arms straight.*
3 *Rest your knees on your upper arms and rock forward, keeping your head up.*
4 *When you feel your weight on your wrists, slowly raise one foot off the ground and then the other. Hold the position. If you cannot lift your feet, just hold the position with your weight on your wrists (Figure 3.14).*

How many/how long: try to hold the crow for at least 5 seconds, gradually increasing the time to 30 seconds. Repeat 2–3 times.

Remember: don't lower your head.

Caution: place a cushion on the ground in front of you, in case you lose your balance.

PEACOCK (FIGURE 3.15)

When you've mastered this pose, your body resembles a beautiful peacock with its feathers spread.

When to do: anytime.

Benefits of the peacock pose
▶ *Tones your digestive system.*
▶ *Brings and maintains the flexibility to your hands, wrists and fingers.*
▶ *Strengthens your forearms and shoulders.*
▶ *Stimulates your solar plexus chakra.*

How to do the peacock pose

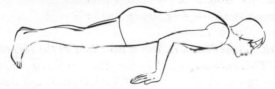

Figure 3.15 The peacock.

1 *Sit on your heels and bring your knees wide apart.*
2 *Bring your elbows, forearms and wrists together in front of your chest with your palms upwards.*
3 *Place the palms of your hands flat on the ground between your knees, with your fingers pointing in towards your body.*
4 *Bend your elbows into your abdomen, without letting your arms move apart.*
5 *Lean forwards and rest your forehead on the ground.*

6 *Stretch one leg straight back and then the other. You are now balancing on your toes, hands and forehead.*

7 *Lift your head so that you are standing on your hands and toes.*

8 *Slowly shift your weight forward until you feel your feet come off the ground (Figure 3.15). DO NOT JUMP!*

How many/how long: hold the peacock for 2–3 seconds, gradually building up to 15 seconds.

Remember: to come into the peacock slowly.

Caution: don't attempt the peacock if you're pregnant, menstruating or experiencing abdominal cramps.

Sitting and forward bending: focusing within

As you bend forward, your view of the physical world around you becomes more defined and focused, encouraging your mind to move inwards. Forward bends require patience, encouraging you to become more tolerant and enduring.

TAILOR – SIMPLE CROSS-LEGGED POSITION (FIGURE 3.16)

This is an easy comfortable pose for pranayama and meditation.

When to do: during pranayama and meditation.

Benefits of the tailor pose
▶ *It provides a firm base for your body, while encouraging both your body and your mind to stay centred.*
▶ *With regular practice, tightness in your hips and lower back is relieved.*
▶ *The muscles of your lower back are strengthened.*

How to do the tailor pose

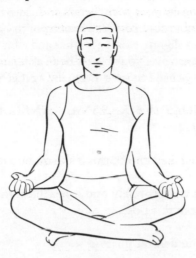

Figure 3.16 The tailor.

1 *Sit in a simple cross-legged position. Check your body to make sure that your head is erect with your chin parallel to the ground, your back is straight and your shoulders are not hunched (Figure 3.16).*
2 *It's important that your knees are no higher than your hips. If you're a beginner or your hips are stiff, it's strongly suggested that you sit on a cushion, block or folded blanket. This will lift your buttocks and bring your hips in line with your knees. It will help to relieve any tension you might be experiencing in your lower back and hips.*
3 *Take a few deep breaths; let your breath settle into a slow natural rhythm.*

How many/how long: sit in this position for as long as you feel comfortable.

Remember: to keep your body relaxed but fully erect.

Caution: if you experience any discomfort in the tailor pose, be sure to use a cushion or block to raise your buttocks.

THUNDERBOLT (VAJRASANA) – KNEELING POSITION (FIGURE 3.17)

If you attend a Zen meditation, this is the traditional sitting position.

When to do: you will probably find it beneficial to practise meditation or eat in this pose.

Benefits of the thunderbolt pose
▶ *Sitting in the thunderbolt pose during or immediately after meals enhances digestion.*
▶ *It stimulates and balances the energy in the region of your solar plexus chakra.*
▶ *The thunderbolt pose offers an alternative meditation position for people who are unable or uncomfortable sitting cross-legged.*

How to do the thunderbolt pose

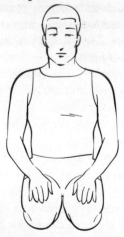

Figure 3.17 The thunderbolt.

1 *Kneel on the ground so that you are sitting with your buttocks resting firmly on your heels. Have your feet together; you may prefer to have the knees together or slightly apart.*
2 *Rest your hands lightly on your thighs. Have your back straight and your head erect.*
3 *Feel as though you are rooting yourself firmly, drawing stability and strength from the ground. Pay particular attention to the pull of gravity and its effects on your body. With practice, you will experience a pleasant heaviness that becomes a feeling of stability and stillness (Figure 3.17).*

How many/how long: sit for as long as you feel comfortable.

Remember: to kneel on a mat or folded blanket. Kneeling benches are also available.

Caution: if you find you're having discomfort in your ankles or feet, you might want to cushion them with a rolled-up face cloth.

LOTUS (FIGURE 3.18)

The lotus is often seen as the signature pose of hatha yoga.

Emerging from the mud and muck the lotus plant grows up through the water, but is unaffected by its environment, i.e. its leaves are water resistant. This most beautiful flower overcomes many physical obstacles in its yearning to reach the light.

When to do: for pranayama, meditation or as a preliminary for certain other advanced asanas.

Benefits of the lotus pose
▶ *Your body is provided with a firm base for meditation and pranayama.*
▶ *Your hips are opened.*

How to do the lotus pose

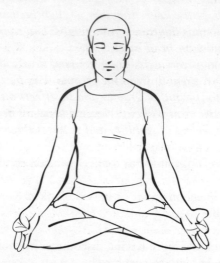

Figure 3.18 The lotus.

1 *Sit with your legs in front of your trunk.*
2 *Bend your right knee and place your right foot as high on your left thigh as possible.*
3 *Then bend your left knee; place your left foot onto your right thigh (Figure 3.18).*

How many/how long: begin by holding for 10 seconds. Gradually increase the time, but hold the pose only as long as you feel absolutely no discomfort.

Remember: to have both knees on the ground.

Caution: the lotus is an advanced yoga pose, requiring a great amount of hip flexibility. Do not try to force your legs into this position. If you have knee problems or varicose veins DO NOT ATTEMPT the lotus pose.

SEATED FORWARD BEND – OR 'WESTERN' STRETCH (FIGURE 3.19)

When you face the rising sun to practise asanas, as recommended by ancient yoga texts, your back is towards the West. The seated forward bend gives an intensive stretch to the entire 'Western' part of your body – from your heels up to your scalp.

When to do: start your forward bending series with this pose.

Benefits of the seated forward bend
▶ *Gives a powerful massage to all of your internal organs.*
▶ *Regular practice relieves compression of the spine.*
▶ *Stretches the hamstrings.*
▶ *Holding this pose for an extended period calms your mind and assists you in becoming more introspective.*

How to do the seated forward bend

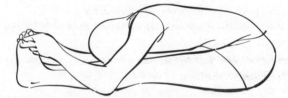

Figure 3.19 Seated forward bend.

1 *Sit up with your legs together and straight out in front of you. Beginners who find this position uncomfortable may want to sit on a block or folded blanket.*
2 *Inhale deeply as you stretch your arms straight up. Have your elbows straight and your arms alongside your ears with your fingers pointing straight upwards.*
3 *Exhale and stretch forward from your hips. Try to keep your back straight.*

4   *If possible, take hold of your feet or ankles. If you cannot reach them, you may want to use a strap – or hold your shins or knees.*
5   *Hold the position and breathe deeply. With each exhalation, feel as though some of the tension is being released from your hips – and sink forward a bit more (Figure 3.19).*

How many/how long: beginners may hold the position for 10 seconds before coming up and repeating the stretch again 2–3 times. As you become more advanced, gradually increase the time to 3 minutes.

Remember: do not arch your back. Feel as though you are stretching forward, not down.

Caution: if you are pregnant, do this pose with your legs apart. It's best to learn this from a teacher who specializes in pregnancy yoga.

INCLINED PLANE (FIGURE 3.20)

An excellent counter-pose to the seated forward bend.

When to do: practise immediately after the seated forward bend.

Benefits of the inclined plane pose
▶ *Strengthens your arms, shoulders and wrists.*
▶ *Promotes flexibility in your spine and hips.*
▶ *Enhances your balance and co-ordination.*

How to do the inclined plane pose

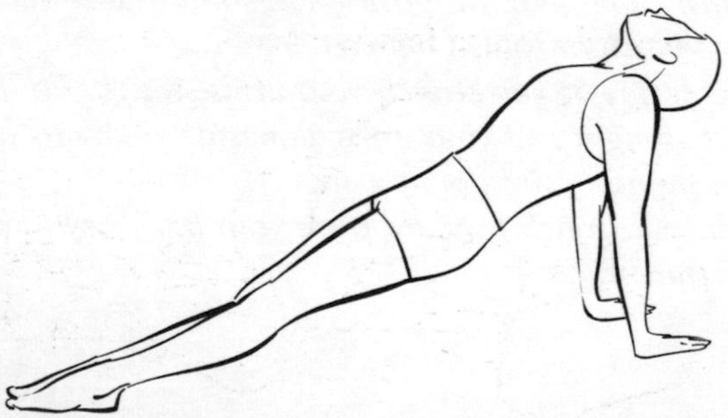

Figure 3.20 Inclined plane.

1 *Sit on the ground with your legs together and straight out in front of you.*

2 *Place your hands flat on the ground behind your back, about 30 cm away from your buttocks. Have your fingers pointing away from your body.*

3 *Drop your head back and lift your hips up as high as you can. Keep your feet together and try to bring them flat onto the ground (Figure 3.20).*
How many/how long: hold for 10 seconds, gradually increasing to 1 minute.

Remember: don't permit your feet to rotate outwards.

Caution: do not attempt if you have carpal tunnel syndrome or are suffering from repetitive strain injury in your wrists/hands.

SINGLE-LEGGED FORWARD BEND (FIGURE 3.21)

This simple variation of the seated forward bend greatly increases hip flexibility.

When to do: do this as a variation after the seated forward bend and inclined plane.

Benefits of the single-legged forward bend

▶ *Stretches and strengthens your entire back.*
▶ *Brings flexibility to your hips.*
▶ *It's an excellent preparatory exercise if you are experiencing physical discomfort when you try to sit for meditation.*

How to do the single-legged forward bend

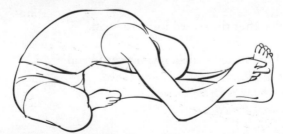

Figure 3.21 Single-legged forward bend.

1 *Sit up with your legs straight out in front of you.*
2 *Bend your right knee and place your right foot next to the inside of your left thigh. Be sure that you do not twist your body to one side as you do this.*
3 *Gently, lower your right knee towards the ground, bringing it down as much as you can without forcing it. Keep your left knee straight.*
4 *Inhale as you lift both of your arms straight up over your head.*
5 *Exhale as you bend forward from your hips. Catch hold of your left foot (use a strap if necessary) and bring your breastbone down towards your left thigh (Figure 3.21). If you are unable to reach your foot, hold onto your shin or your left knee.*
6 *Breathe deeply as you hold the position, and then inhale as you stretch your body up to the starting position. Repeat the pose on the other side.*

How many/how long: try to remain in the position for 10–30 seconds, gradually increase the time until you are holding the position for 1 minute.

Remember: come down straight; do not permit your body to twist.

Caution: do not try to force your knee down to the ground.

SEATED WIDE-ANGLE FORWARD BEND (FIGURE 3.22)

A forward bend that stretches the hard-to-reach inner thighs.

When to do: after the seated forward bend.

Benefits of the seated wide-angle forward bend
▶ *Inner thighs are stretched and toned.*
▶ *Lower back is strengthened.*
▶ *Hips are opened.*

How to do the seated wide-angle forward bend

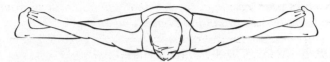

Figure 3.22 Seated wide-angle forward bend.

1 *Sit with your legs as wide apart as possible and your knees straight.*
2 *Turn to face your right leg.*
3 *Breathe in deeply as you stretch your arms straight up over your head.*
4 *Exhale as you lean forward and come down onto your right leg.*
5 *Hold the pose, breathing deeply. Inhale up.*
6 *Repeat steps 2–5 on your left side.*
7 *Bring your body to the centre and exhale as you bend straight down. Catch hold of both legs with the respective hands and drop your head towards the ground (Figure 3.22). Breathe deeply as you hold the position; inhale up.*

How many/how long: hold for 10 seconds on each side, gradually increasing to 1 minute.

Remember: to relax into the pose. Hold the position and focus on your breath.

Caution: do not use force to pull your body downwards.

BUTTERFLY – AND BOUND-ANGLE POSE (FIGURE 3.23)

This pose is actually two exercises in one. When you flutter your knees, it's known as the butterfly. When you hold still and practise it as a static pose, it's known as the bound angle.

When to do: after the seated wide-angle forward bend.

Benefits of the butterfly and bound-angle pose

▶ *Opens your hips.*
▶ *Relaxes your legs.*
▶ *Relieves tension around the knees and ankles.*

How to do the butterfly and bound-angle pose

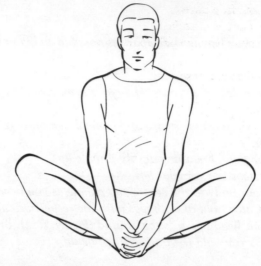

Figure 3.23 The butterfly and bound-angle.

1 *Sit on the ground, bend your knees and bring the soles of your feet together. Bring your knees out towards the sides and allow them to drop towards the ground.*
2 *Hold your feet together with your hands and gently bounce your knees up and down, trying to bring your knees as close to the ground as possible. This is the butterfly (Figure 3.23).*
3 *When your hips feel sufficiently loosened, try the bound-angle. Keep your knees still, hold your soles together and gently lower your chest towards your feet.*

How many/how long: sit for about 30 seconds, bouncing your knees in the butterfly. If you are a beginner, do only this much. More advanced students can attempt the bound-angle pose and hold it for 10–30 seconds.

Remember: do not force your knees down.

FROG (FIGURE 3.24)

In this pose, your body resembles a frog about to leap.

When to do: with your other forward bending poses.

Benefits of the frog pose
▶ *Lower back is stretched.*
▶ *Chest, shoulders and hips are opened.*

How to do the frog pose

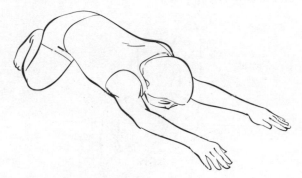

Figure 3.24 The frog.

1 *Sit on your heels in thunderbolt (pages 64–65). Bring your knees wide apart.*
2 *Place your hands to the ground between your knees.*
3 *Slowly walk your hands forward, keeping your buttocks on your heels.*
4 *Continue walking forward until your chest is on the ground (or as close as is comfortably possible) and your arms are stretched straight out on either side of your head (Figure 3.24).*
5 *Breathe deeply and hold the pose.*

How many/how long: hold for 10 seconds, gradually increasing to 30 seconds.

Remember: to keep your buttocks on your heels.

COW'S HEAD (FIGURE 3.25)

In this pose your elbow resembles the horn of an Indian cow.

When to do: as part of your seated poses.

Benefits of the cow's head pose
▶ *Stretches your shoulders.*
▶ *Prepares your body for more advanced asanas.*
▶ *Stretches the side muscles on either side of the rib cage.*

How to do the cow's head pose

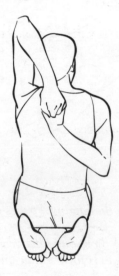

Figure 3.25 The cow's head.

1 *Sit on your heels in thunderbolt (page 64).*
2 *Bend your right elbow; bring your right hand behind your back.*
3 *Bend your left elbow and bring it up over your shoulder, with your hand hanging down towards your shoulder.*
4 *Clasp your hands together behind your back (Figure 3.25).*
5 *If your hands don't reach each other, hold a strap or face cloth in your upper hand. Reach back with your other hand and hold the strap or cloth. Bring your hands as close together as you can.*

6 *With your hands in this position, take a deep breath and try to bring your head to the ground in front of you.*
7 *Breathe as you hold the pose. Inhale as you sit up and repeat on the other side with the left elbow behind your back and the right up over your shoulder.*

How many/how long: hold for 10 seconds, gradually increasing to 30 seconds.

Remember: if you can't clasp your hands together, use a strap or a folded face cloth.

LION (FIGURE 3.26)

If you are practising asanas with children, be sure to include the lion pose.

When to do: anytime.

Benefits of the lion pose
▶ *Brings energy to your neck and throat region.*

How to do the lion pose

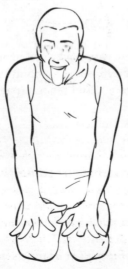

Figure 3.26 The lion.

1 *Sit on your heels in thunderbolt (page 64). Rest the palms of your hands on your thighs with your fingers extended.*

2 *Inhale deeply and exhale strongly through your mouth. As you exhale, 'spring' forward like a lion about to jump on its prey: straighten your arms, stiffen your body, make 'claws' of your fingers, stick your tongue out as far as possible and bulge your eyes (Figure 3.26).*

How many/how long: 2–3 times.

Remember: roaring sounds are optional, but much appreciated by young friends!

Back bends: opening up to the world

Back bends stretch your spine in a backward direction. They open your chest, release your hips and counteract the effects of sitting at a desk/computer all day. Among the different types of asanas, back bends are the most extroverted. They are more vigorous to practise and help you to open up to the wonder of the world around you.

BRIDGE (FIGURE 3.27)

The bridge is a relatively easy backward bending pose that helps to create an experience of expansion, in contrast to the introversion of the shoulderstand (page 97) and plough (page 99).

When to do: after the shoulderstand.

Benefits of the bridge
▶ *The bridge is a counter-stretch to the shoulderstand.*
▶ *It relieves pressure from your cervical region (neck and upper back).*
▶ *Your abdominal and lumbar (lower back) muscles are strengthened.*
▶ *It encourages flexibility of your wrists and spine.*

How to do the bridge pose

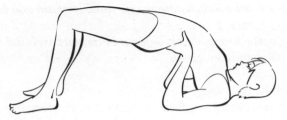

Figure 3.27 The bridge.

1 *Lie flat on your back.*
2 *Bend your knees and bring your feet flat onto the floor. Have your feet parallel and hip-width apart.*
3 *Lift your hips as high as possible.*
4 *Place your hands flat onto your back with your fingers pointing in towards your spine and your thumbs up towards ceiling (Figure 3.27).*
5 *Come down and relax for a moment.*

How many/how long: hold the bridge for about 1 minute, breathing deeply. If you are doing the half-wheel variation, hold the pose for 10–30 seconds, but repeat it 2–3 times.

Remember: don't permit your feet to turn outward; keep your knees in line with your feet.

VARIATIONS OF THE BRIDGE

Variation 1
Extend your arms on the ground under your body. Interlock your fingers, keeping your elbows straight.

Variation 2
Also known as the half-wheel. Hold each of your ankles with the respective hand. This variation may be done just before the full-wheel (page 87). If you are not able to come into the wheel, practise this variation of the bridge to prepare your body.

FISH (FIGURE 3.28)

This is the second counter-pose to the shoulderstand and plough.

When to do: the fish is usually done immediately after the shoulderstand and plough.

Benefits of the fish pose

▶ *The pose opens your chest so that your breathing is enhanced. If you tend to breathe shallowly, have panic attacks and/ or have asthma, you will probably find that regular practice of the fish helps to strengthen your respiratory system so that you can overcome your breathing problems. However, never attempt to do asanas when you are actually having an asthmatic attack.*

▶ *Your shoulders are stretched back; this is an excellent pose if you tend to have rounded shoulders and/or sit at a computer all day.*

▶ *The fish helps to increase the energy to your neck and shoulder area.*

How to do the fish pose

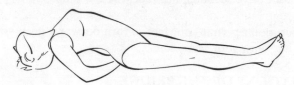

Figure 3.28 The fish.

1 *Lie flat on your back with your legs out straight. Bring your legs and feet together.*
2 *Place your hands, palms downward, under your respective buttocks/thighs.*
3 *Bend your elbows, pushing them into the ground. Arch your chest upward and place the top of your head gently onto the floor. Hold the position, with your weight mainly on your elbows. There should be very little weight on your head or neck (Figure 3.28).*

4 *Your chest is wide open in this position, so take advantage of it by breathing as deeply as possible. Be sure to engage your rib cage in the breathing. Imagine that your ribs are like the gills of a fish, opening to pull oxygen and prana into your body.*

5 *To come out of the position: lift your head slightly, slide your head back and lower your back to the ground. After the fish, remember to relax for a few moments in the corpse pose (page 110).*

How many/how long: hold the fish pose for approximately 30 seconds and then come down to relax on the ground. Gradually build up to 2 minutes.

Remember: to have your weight on your elbows. There should be no pressure on your head or neck.

Caution: do not do the fish if you have a whiplash or other recent neck injury, high blood pressure or suffer from migraine headaches.

COBRA (FIGURE 3.29)

Begin by tuning into the vibrant energy of the king of snakes, which coils itself up and back.

When to do: at the beginning of your backward bending series.

BENEFITS OF THE COBRA POSE

▶ *Enhances general flexibility of your spine and back muscles.*
▶ *Helps to relieve hunched shoulders and a rounded back.*
▶ *Massages, tones and strengthens your back muscles, particularly in your lumbar region.*
▶ *With practice, the range of motion in your spine increases.*
▶ *Massages internal abdominal organs.*

HOW TO DO THE COBRA POSE

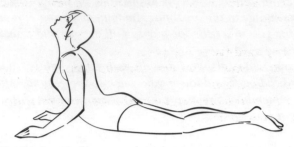

Figure 3.29 The cobra.

1 Lie on your front, face downwards. Place your hands flat on the ground, directly beneath your shoulders. Have your fingertips in line with your shoulders.
2 Visualizing the upward coiling movement of a cobra, begin to slowly roll up and back as much as possible.
3 Keep your abdomen on the ground. Allow your elbows to remain slightly bent and in towards your sides (Figure 3.29).
4 Breathe deeply and hold the position. When you are ready, come down by slowly uncoiling your body.
   How many/how long: beginners may hold for 10 seconds; repeat 2–3 times. As you advance, try to extend the time you hold the cobra to 30 seconds.
   Remember: to keep your shoulders relaxed – down and away from your ears.

Caution: don't attempt the cobra if you're pregnant. However, there are many excellent backward-bending alternatives, which are best learned from a teacher who specializes in pregnancy yoga.

UPWARD-FACING DOG (FIGURE 3.30)

In this pose, which is sometimes confused with the cobra, you lift most of your body off the ground, supporting yourself on your hands and the tops of your feet.

When to do: before or after downward-facing dog (page 42) or as a transition asana, moving between forward bends and/or standing poses.

Benefits of upward-facing dog pose
▶ *Strengthens your wrists, arms and shoulders.*
▶ *Opens your chest.*
▶ *Stretches your lumbar region without putting pressure on any part of your spine.*

How to do upward-facing dog pose

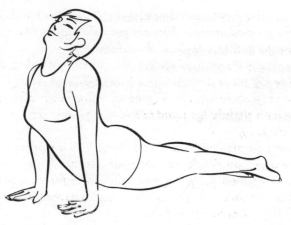

Figure 3.30 Upward-facing dog.

1 *Lie on your front and place your hands flat on the ground under your shoulders.*
2 *Straighten your arms, which lifts your chest, hips and legs off the ground. Push yourself up until you're resting only on the tops of your feet and your hands. Slide your hips towards your hands.*
3 *Hold the pose with your knees and elbows straight. Feel your shoulders up near your ears (Figure 3.30).*
4 *Hold the position and breathe deeply. Feel how your lower back is hanging.*

How many/how long: beginners may hold for 10 seconds; repeat 2–3 times. As you advance, try to extend the time you hold to 30 seconds.

Remember: to have the tops of your feet on the ground.

Caution: be careful with this pose if you have wrist problems.

HALF-LOCUST (FIGURE 3.31)

This pose is sometimes referred to as the grasshopper.

When to do: after the cobra, but before the locust.

Benefits of the half-locust pose
▶ *Strengthens your lower back.*
▶ *Brings flexibility to your upper spine (cervical region).*

How to do the half-locust pose

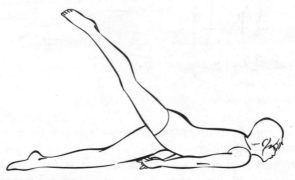

Figure 3.31 *The half-locust.*

1 *Lie on your front with your arms straight beside your body.*
2 *Bring your arms beneath your body and interlock your fingers, keeping your elbows straight.*
3 *Stretch your neck forward and place your chin on the ground.*
4 *Inhale as you lift your right leg. Exhale as you replace your leg on the ground (Figure 3.31).*
5 *Repeat on left side.*

How many/how long: repeat this 2–3 times on each side, holding for 10 seconds and gradually building up to 30 seconds.

Remember: ensure that your hips remain straight as you lift each leg. Keep your chin on the ground.

Caution: don't attempt the half-locust if you're pregnant.

LOCUST (FIGURE 3.32)

If you find it uncomfortable to keep your hands under your body in the half-locust and locust, try doing these poses with your hands next to your body. Have your elbows straight and your palms on the ground, next to your hips.

When to do: immediately after the half-locust.

Benefits of the locust pose
▶ *Stretches the cervical (neck and upper back) region of your spine.*
▶ *Strengthens the lumbar (lower back) region.*
▶ *Massages your internal organs.*
▶ *Strengthens your arm muscles.*

How to do the locust pose

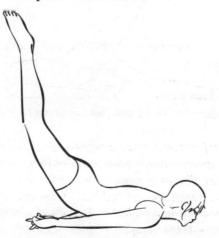

Figure 3.32 The locust.

1 *Lie on your front with your arms straight alongside your body.*
2 *Bring your arms beneath your body and interlock your fingers, keeping your elbows straight.*
3 *Stretch your neck forward and place your chin on the ground.*
4 *Take three deep breaths to prepare yourself physically and mentally for practising the locust. On the third inhalation, slowly lift both legs off the ground as high as you can (Figure 3.32). If you are a beginner, you may only be able to lift a few centimetres. However, with regular practice, you will improve rapidly.*
5 *Hold this position and breathe. Then slowly replace both legs on the ground.*

How many/how long: hold for 3–5 seconds, gradually building up to 30 seconds. Repeat 2–3 times.

Remember: make sure that you keep your chin on the ground.

Caution: don't attempt the locust if you're pregnant.

BOW (FIGURE 3.33)

The bow combines many of the benefits of the cobra and locust poses.

When to do: practising the bow after the cobra and/or locust poses, enhances the benefits.

Benefits of the bow pose
▶ *A comprehensive backward bend is given to your entire spine and all the back muscles.*
▶ *Your internal organs are massaged.*
▶ *If you sit at a computer all day and/or have a tendency to hunch your shoulders, the bow will help to counteract the negative effects.*
▶ *Your chest is expanded; this is of particular benefit if you suffer from asthma or other respiratory problems.*

How to do the bow pose

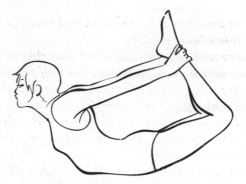

Figure 3.33 The bow.

1 *Lie face downwards on your abdomen.*
2 *Bend your knees and bring your feet up.*
3 *Reach back and take hold of your ankles. If you are unable to reach, place a yoga strap or small towel around your ankles and hold on to that.*
4 *Keeping your elbows straight, inhale as you lift your head, chest and legs off the ground. Lift your legs as high as possible (Figure 3.33). Breathe as you hold the position. Then return your body to the ground.*
5 *Relax for a few seconds and then come up into the bow again.*

How many/how long: try to do the bow 2–3 times, holding for 10 seconds each time. You may find that you can gradually build up to holding for 30 seconds each time.

Remember: to keep your elbows straight.

Caution: don't attempt the bow if you are pregnant.

BOAT (FIGURE 3.34)

If you're unable to hold your ankles in the bow, this pose is an alternative. However, its effect is more to strengthen your back muscles than to bring flexibility.

When to do: the boat may be practised in place of the bow – after either the cobra or locust poses.

Benefits of the boat pose
- ▶ *Strengthens your back muscles.*
- ▶ *Massages your internal organs.*

How to do the boat pose

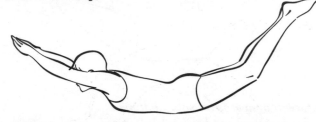

Figure 3.34 The boat.

1 *Lie face downwards on your abdomen.*
2 *Stretch your arms straight out in front of you, trying to keep them next to your ears. Keep your legs straight.*
3 *Inhale as you lift your arms, head, chest and legs off the ground as high as possible (Figure 3.34). Breathe as you hold the position.*
4 *Come down, relax for a few seconds and then come into the boat pose again.*

How many/how long: try to hold for 10 seconds, gradually increasing to 30 seconds. Do this 2–3 times.

Remember: to keep your arms straight and next to your ears.

Caution: don't attempt the boat if you're pregnant.

WHEEL (FIGURE 3.35)

The wheel gives a full backward bend to your spine. Your entire body is facing outward, which can be very conducive to expansive consciousness.

When to do: at the end of your backward bending series.

Benefits of the wheel pose
▶ *The wheel gives your body the optimum benefits of all backward bending poses.*
▶ *It strengthens your arms while bringing an increase of flexibility to your spine.*
▶ *It opens your hips and chest.*

How to do the wheel pose

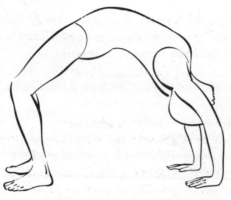

Figure 3.35 The wheel.

1 *Lie flat on your back with your knees bent and your feet flat on the ground. Try to have your feet parallel to each other and as close to your buttocks as possible.*
2 *Place your palms flat on the ground behind your shoulders, with your fingers pointing in towards your body.*
3 *Lift your hips, then your chest. Bring the top of your head to the ground.*
4 *Straighten your arms as you arch your hips and chest upwards. Only your hands and feet are now on the ground (Figure 3.35).*
5 *Breathe deeply as you hold the position. Then lower your back to the ground and relax.*

How many/how long: try to hold for at least 10 seconds, gradually building up to 30 seconds. You may repeat this 2–3 times.

Remember: to keep your feet parallel to each other.

Caution: the wheel is not suggested if you have high blood pressure or glaucoma. Be careful when attempting it if you have had wrist or shoulder injuries.

CAMEL (FIGURE 3.36)

The camel is sometimes referred to as the seated wheel. Although it gives many of the benefits of an extreme backward bend, the camel doesn't require the same strength to practise.

When to do: at the end of your backward bending series, in place of the wheel.

Benefits of the camel pose
- ▶ *An integral backward bend for your spine and back muscles.*
- ▶ *An excellent hip opener.*

How to do the camel pose

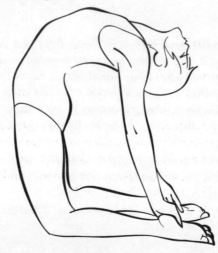

Figure 3.36 The camel.

1 *Sit on your heels in the thunderbolt pose (see page 64).*
2 *Lift your hips and trunk so that you are standing on your knees. It's best to have your knees together, but you may let them separate slightly, if necessary. Have your knees and feet the same distance apart from each other.*
3 *Reach back with your right hand and catch hold of your right heel. Then reach with your left hand to hold on to your left heel. If you have difficulty in reaching your heels, place your hands flat on the floor behind your feet.*
4 *Let your head drop back. Lift your hips up and forward as much as possible. Feel your breastbone arching up towards the sky (Figure 3.36).*
5 *Breathe deeply as you hold the pose.*

How many/how long: try to hold the camel for 10 seconds, gradually increasing the time to 30 seconds. Come down; relax in the child's pose (page 112). Repeat 2–3 times.

Remember: breathe as you hold the camel pose.

Caution: people with knee or neck injuries should be especially careful when attempting the camel.

Twists: wringing out negativity

Twisting poses rotate your body while squeezing out physical impurities and mental tension. Practise only one of the following twisting poses; they are listed according to their difficulty. Start with the first and work up to the most difficult. On days when you're feeling particularly stiff or blocked, retreat a step or two. In yoga it's often a good idea to go back to the basics. The rotated triangle (pages 50–51) is also an excellent twist – and the triangle gives a very good lateral stretch to your body.

SIMPLE SPINAL TWIST (FIGURE 3.37)

If you're a beginner, feel stiff or if you're pregnant, practise this
simple variation of the twist.

When to do: after both backward and forward bending.

Benefits of the simple spinal twist
▶ *Maintains flexibility between the vertebrae.*
▶ *Massages your internal organs.*

How to do the simple spinal twist

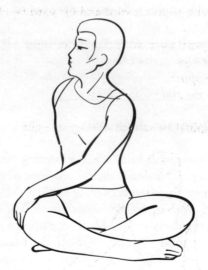

Figure 3.37 *Simple spinal twist.*

1 *Sit in a simple cross-legged position (page 63).*
2 *Place your right hand on your left knee and your left hand behind your back – on the ground or on a block (Figure 3.37). Twist your upper body to the left; look over your left shoulder.*
3 *Breathe as you hold the pose. Make sure that your spine is perpendicular to the ground and your head is level.*
4 *Release the position and repeat on the other side.*

How many/how long: hold the pose for 10 seconds on each side, gradually increasing to 30 seconds.

Remember: to keep your back at a right angle to the ground.

SPINAL TWIST WITH ONE LEG STRAIGHT (FIGURE 3.38)

Still a fairly simple pose.

When to do: after both backward and forward bending.

Benefits of the spinal twist with one leg straight
▶ *Opens your hips.*
▶ *Aligns your spine.*
▶ *Massages your abdominal organs.*

How to do the spinal twist with one leg straight

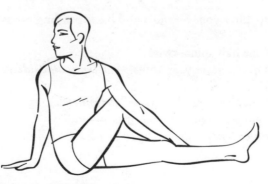

Figure 3.38 Spinal twist with one leg straight.

1 *Sit on the ground with your legs straight out in front of you.*
2 *Bend your right knee and bring your right leg over your left. Place your right foot flat on the ground with your right knee up.*
3 *Twist to the right. Bring your left arm to the outside of your right knee. Push against your right knee with your left elbow.*
4 *Place your right hand on the floor behind your back; try to keep your spine upright (Figure 3.38). Don't lean over. If you are unable to reach the floor, use a block.*
5 *Release the position and repeat on the other side.*

How many/how long: hold the pose for 10 seconds on each side, gradually increasing to 30 seconds.

Remember: to keep your back straight.

Caution: don't attempt this pose when you're pregnant. This pose is a bit easier than the half-spinal twist. It's suggested that you perfect the easier position first before attempting the next, more difficult, ones.

HALF SPINAL TWIST (FIGURE 3.39)

The Sanskrit name for this pose is ardha-matsyendrasana, named after one of the first teachers of hatha yoga.

When to do: after your forward and back bending poses.

Benefits of the half spinal twist
▶ *Helps to maintain your spine's elasticity and side-to-side mobility.*
▶ *Gives a lateral stretch to your back muscles.*
▶ *Massages the organs in your abdomen.*
▶ *Stimulates and purifies your solar plexus chakra.*

How to do the half spinal twist

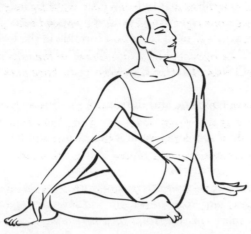

Figure 3.39 Half spinal twist.

1 *Come into a kneeling position, sitting on your heels.*
2 *Drop your hips to the floor on the right side of your feet.*
3 *Place your left foot flat on the floor outside of your right knee, with your left knee up.*
4 *Stretch your right arm up; bring it over and around your left knee.*
5 *Try to hold your left ankle with your right hand. If you can't reach your left ankle, hold onto your right knee (the knee on the ground). Look over your left shoulder (Figure 3.39).*
6 *Breathe deeply as you hold this pose. With each exhalation, feel that you are going more deeply into it.*
7 *Release the position and repeat on the other side.*

How many/how long: hold for 10 seconds on each side; gradually increase the time you hold this pose to 30 seconds on each side.

Remember: to keep both buttocks on the ground.

Caution: don't attempt this pose when you're pregnant. There are a number of variations that don't put pressure on your abdomen, but these are best learned from a teacher who specializes in pregnancy yoga. Also be careful of this pose if you have had a hip replacement.

Insight

There is also a full spinal twist. We have not included it in this book, as it is a very advanced position. Before you attempt it, you will need to be comfortable in the lotus pose.

SAGE'S TWIST (FIGURE 3.40)

This is the most energetic and difficult of the twisting poses.

When to do: do a simpler twist first before attempting this one.

Benefits of the sage's twist
- ▶ *Deeply massages your internal organs.*
- ▶ *Brings flexibility to both the hip and shoulder regions.*
- ▶ *Focuses energy in your solar plexus region.*

How to do the sage's twist

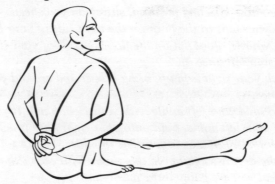

Figure 3.40 Sage's twist.

1 *Sit on the ground with your legs straight out in front of you.*
2 *Bend your right knee and bring it close to your chest. Place your right foot flat on the ground with your heel as close to your trunk as possible.*
3 *Turn to your left. Stretch your right arm forward inside your right knee. Bring your arm around your right knee.*

4 *Bring your left hand behind your back. Try to take hold of your left wrist with your right hand (Figure 3.40). If you are unable to reach, use a strap.*
5 *Hold the pose and breathe deeply. Then release and try it on the other side.*

How many/how long: hold for 10 seconds on each side, gradually building up to 30 seconds.

Remember: to breathe as you hold the position.

Caution: don't attempt this pose when you're pregnant.

Advanced variation
Keeping hold of your wrist, try to bring your chin down to your left knee.

RECLINING SPINAL TWIST (FIGURE 3.41)

This is a very simple, but effective, spinal twist for whenever you feel a bit stiff and/or tense.

When to do: any time your lower back feels tense; after both backward and forward bending.

Benefits of the reclining spinal twist
▶ *Releases tension in your lower back.*
▶ *Gently stretches your shoulders.*

How to do the reclining spinal twist

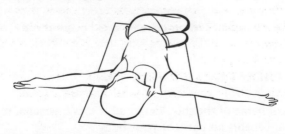

Figure 3.41 Reclining spinal twist.

1 *Lie on your back. Stretch your arms out to the side on the floor at shoulder level.*
2 *Bend your knees up towards your chest.*
3 *Bring your knees to the floor to the right of your body.*
4 *Turn your head and look at your left hand, which is still stretched out on the ground at shoulder level (Figure 3.41).*
5 *Hold the pose; return to centre and repeat steps 2–4 on your left side.*

How many/how long: hold the pose 10 seconds on each side, gradually increasing to 30 seconds.

Remember: to try to keep your hips on the ground as much as possible.

Inverted poses: attain a new vision of life

Turning yourself upside down offers interesting opportunities for you to enhance your views of life. To maintain your inverted position, you must be fully present in the here and now. The movement of your head is more limited and your line of sight is more concentrated. You become more aware of yourself as the one who is witnessing and less open to distractions from the outside world. Your arms and shoulder girdle take on the functions that your legs and hips normally perform.

Inverted poses encourage lightness of thought as well as grace in your physical body.

Women are advised not to practise inverted poses during menstruation.

SHOULDERSTAND (FIGURE 3.42)

The Sanskrit name of the shoulderstand is sarvangasana, meaning 'a pose that benefits all parts of your body'.

When to do: some schools of yoga practise the shoulderstand at the beginning of their asana session. Other traditions believe that it's better to use it as a cool-down pose at the end.

Benefits of the shoulderstand

▶ *As you hold the pose, you will notice how your chin presses on your throat. The shoulderstand strengthens and balances your thyroid gland, which is located at your neck. Your thyroid controls metabolism and other endocrine glands.*

▶ *It helps to drain stagnant blood from your lower extremities.*

▶ *The cervical region of your spine is stretched, as well as your shoulder and upper back muscles.*

▶ *Energy is focused on your throat chakra.*

▶ *The shoulderstand helps to relieve your mental lethargy.*

How to do the shoulderstand

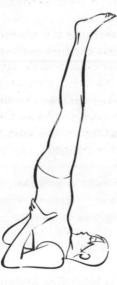

Figure 3.42 The shoulderstand.

1 *Lie on your back. Be sure that you are at least 1.5 metres away from the wall. Bring your legs together and raise them to a 90-degree angle.*

2 *Bring your hands onto your buttocks. Slowly walk your hands along your back, using your hands to raise and support your back. Lift yourself up until you are as straight as possible. Try to have your hands flat on your back, with your fingers pointing in towards your spine and thumbs around the side and towards the front (Figure 3.42).*

3 *Consciously relax your calves and your feet. Hold the position.*

4 *From the shoulderstand, you can choose to either come down or come into the plough pose (see opposite).*

5 *When coming down, drop your legs halfway back to the ground; bring your hands flat on the floor.*

6 *Making sure to keep your head down, slowly unroll your body, bringing each vertebra to the ground separately.*

How many/how long: if you are a beginner, hold the shoulderstand for no more than 10 seconds. As you start to feel comfortable in the pose, gradually increase the time until you are holding it for 3 minutes.

Remember: to do the plough and the shoulderstand together.

Caution: it's best to avoid the shoulderstand if you have had whiplash or suffer from neck injuries. Don't practise the shoulderstand or any other inverted poses if you are menstruating. If you're more than four months pregnant, you may be able to practise a half-shoulderstand variation. This is best learned from a teacher who specializes in pregnancy yoga.

PLOUGH (FIGURE 3.43)

The plough is an excellent pose for stretching your entire spine; its particular focus is on your neck and shoulders.

When to do: immediately after the shoulderstand and before the bridge (page 77) and fish (page 78).

Benefits of the plough pose

▶ *Your spine is fully stretched.*
▶ *Regular practice of the plough slows the ageing process of your spine.*
▶ *Insomnia is relieved.*
▶ *Your mind becomes calmer and clearer.*
▶ *It greatly enhances the flexibility of your cervical region: neck, upper back and shoulders.*

How to do the plough pose

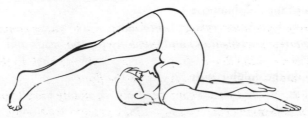

Figure 3.43 The plough.

1 *From the shoulderstand, exhale as you drop one foot to the ground behind your head. Inhale as you raise your leg back to the vertical position. Repeat with your other leg.*
2 *Next, bring both feet to the ground behind your head. Try to get your toes to touch the floor.*
3 *If your feet reach the ground, bring your hands onto the ground behind your back, palms down (Figure 3.43). If your feet can't reach the floor, keep your hands on your back for support.*
4 *Breathe as you hold the plough. When you are ready, slowly roll out of the pose, lowering each vertebra separately while keeping your head on the ground.*

How many/how long: try to hold the plough for 10 seconds, gradually building up to 1 minute.

Remember: to come out of the plough pose slowly, with full control.

Caution: don't attempt the plough if you're pregnant or menstruating. If you have kyphosis (outward curvature) of the spine, don't try to force yourself into this pose; just do as much as you comfortably can.

DOLPHIN (FIGURE 3.44)

This helps you to prepare your arms and shoulders for the headstand.

When to do: the dolphin is best done just before, or in place of, the headstand.

Benefits of the dolphin pose
- ▶ *Strengthens your arms and shoulders.*
- ▶ *Prepares you physically and mentally for the headstand.*

How to do the dolphin pose

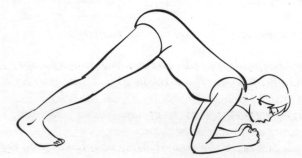

Figure 3.44a The dolphin – chin forward.

1 *Sit on your heels with your knees and feet together.*
2 *Hold the opposite elbow with each of your hands. Place your elbows on the ground so that they are directly under your shoulders.*
3 *Without moving your elbows, release your hands. Clasp your hands together in front of you by interlocking your fingers. Your forearms now form a tripod on the ground.*
4 *Keep your head up and straighten your knees.*
5 *Without moving your arms or feet, rock your body forward so that your chin is in front of your hands (Figure 3.44a).*
6 *Then push your body up and back as far as possible (Figure 3.44b).*

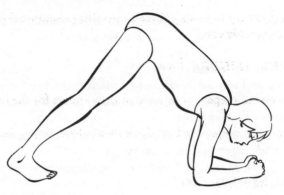

Figure 3.44b. The dolphin – chin back.

How many/how long: rock forward and back 8–10 times. Relax in the child's pose (see page 112) for a few moments – and then try the dolphin again.

Remember: to keep your weight on your elbows.

Caution: if your arms are very weak and you're unable to move forward and back, practise only steps 1–4.

HEADSTAND (FIGURE 3.45)

Often referred to as the 'king of the asanas', the headstand seems to be viewed either with apprehension or as a tonic for a vast range of human ills: physical, mental and spiritual. With regular practice, the headstand brings an abundance of radiant energy to your head and upper body.

Practising the headstand is physically not as difficult as you might imagine; be sure that you have perfected the dolphin before attempting it. For many people the headstand requires more than physical strength; its practice involves facing and overcoming a variety of fears and self-imposed limitations.

When to do: any time that you're feeling tired and in need of a burst of positive energy. Some schools of yoga teach the headstand at the beginning of the asana session. In other traditions, people prefer to do it at the end, as a cool-down technique.

Benefits of the headstand

▶ *Gives a rest to your heart and circulatory system by inverting the body and allowing gravity to assist in the venous return of the blood to your heart.*

▶ *Encourages a slow rate of respiration, while strengthening your respiratory and circulatory systems.*

▶ *Your brain, spinal cord and sympathetic nervous system receive an increase of blood rich in nutrients.*

▶ *Brings lightness to your step and posture.*

▶ *Helps to drain stagnant blood from your lower extremities.*

▶ *Counteracts the pull of gravity on your abdominal and facial muscles.*

▶ *Brings an increased supply of blood to your head, face and neck.*

▶ *Helps you to calm your mind.*

▶ *Memory tends to improve.*

▶ *Self-confidence and empathy increases.*

▶ *You have a greater sense of 'groundedness' in life.*

▶ *Your view of the world is enhanced.*

How to do the headstand

1 *Sit on your heels with your knees and feet together.*

2 *Bend your elbows and place them on the ground so that they are directly under your shoulders. Hold the opposite elbow with each of your hands (Figure 3.45a).*

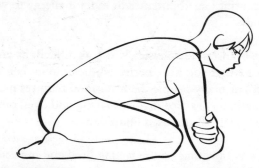

Figure 3.45a The headstand.

3 *Without moving your elbows, release your hands. Clasp your hands together in front of you by interlocking your fingers. Your forearms now form a tripod on the ground. When you perform the headstand with your arms in this tripod position, the weight of your body is on your elbows rather than on your head or neck (Figure 3.45b).*

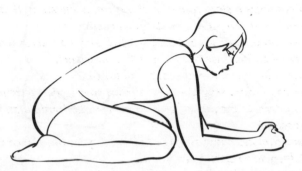

Figure 3.45b.

4 *Place the frontal portion of your head on the ground. Have the back of your head resting gently against your clasped hands (Figure 3.45c).*

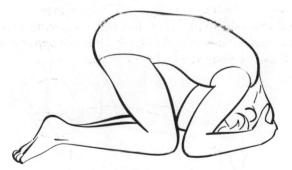

Figure 3.45c.

5 *Straighten your knees without moving your head or elbows (Figure 3.45d).*

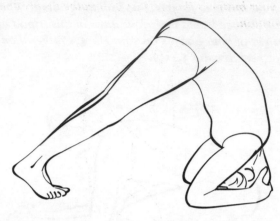

Figure 3.45d.

6 *Slowly walk your feet forward until your hips are directly over your head. Don't allow your arms or head to move as you do this. Make sure that your weight remains on your elbows – don't allow your weight to come onto your head (Figure 3.45e).*

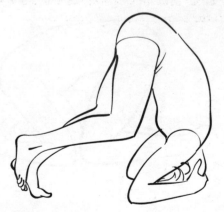

Figure 3.45e.

7 *Bend your knees without letting your hips drop. This will involve you bringing your feet off the floor. Bring your heels up to your buttocks (Figure 3.45f). Breathe deeply and hold this position.*

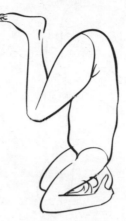

Figure 3.45f.

This is known as the half-headstand. Make sure that you can comfortably hold it for at least 10 seconds before going any further in attempting the full headstand.

8 *Keep your knees bent and together as you slowly bring them up towards the ceiling (Figure 3.45g).*

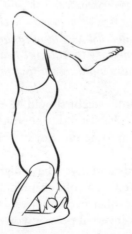

Figure 3.45g.

9 *Straighten your knees, lifting your feet until your body is in a straight line. Have your weight evenly balanced on your elbows (Figure 3.45h).*

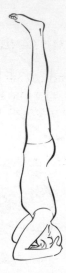

Figure 3.45h.

10 *Breathe deeply and hold the position for as long as you feel comfortable. Be particularly aware of your relationship to gravity.*
11 *When you are ready, come down slowly. Keep your head down and sit back on your heels in the child's pose (see page 112) for at least 2–3 minutes before sitting up. How many/how long: try to hold the headstand for 30 seconds, gradually building up to 3 minutes.*

Remember: that very little weight should be on your head and/or neck. If you're doing the headstand properly, your elbows will be holding you up and supporting most of your weight.

Caution: avoid the headstand if you have high blood pressure, glaucoma, a detached retina, a cold or a blocked nose, or suffer from whiplash or other neck injuries. Don't practise the headstand or any other inverted poses if you're menstruating.

An adapted headstand may be done up until your fourth month of pregnancy, but this is best learned from a teacher who specializes in pregnancy yoga. Don't attempt the headstand in later stages of pregnancy.

SCORPION – FOREARM STAND (FIGURE 3.46)

The scorpion is an advanced pose requiring intensive mental focus and upper-back flexibility. Be sure that you have perfected the headstand, and can hold it comfortably for at least 3 minutes, before attempting the scorpion.

When to do: after you have held the headstand for about 3 minutes.

Benefits of the scorpion
- *Enhances your sense of balance.*
- *Strengthens your arms.*
- *Brings great flexibility to your shoulders and upper back.*

How to do the scorpion pose
1. *Come into the headstand (see Figures 3.45a–h).*
2. *Bend your knees and arch backward, making sure that your weight remains on your elbows (Figure 3.46a).*

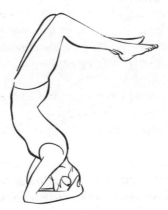

Figure 3.46a The scorpion.

3 *Release the interlocking of your fingers and bring your hands flat onto the ground. Try to have your forearms as parallel as possible (Figure 3.46b).*

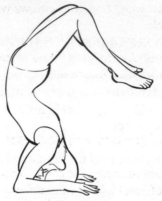

Figure 3.46b.

4 *Lift up from your shoulders, bringing your upper arms perpendicular to the ground. Try to have your shoulders directly over your elbows. Look up, as much as possible (Figure 3.46c).*

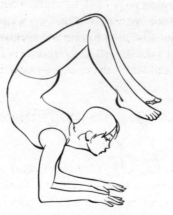

Figure 3.46c.

5 *To come out of the pose: bring your hands together, straighten your legs and come back to the headstand. Come down slowly and relax in the child's pose (page 112) for at least 1 minute before sitting up.*

How many/how long: start with 10 seconds and gradually build up to 1 minute.

Remember: keep your weight on your elbows with your shoulders back as far as possible.

Caution: don't attempt the scorpion if you're menstruating, pregnant or suffer from neck injuries.

Relaxation techniques: winding down

Relaxed muscles function more efficiently and stretch further. There's less chance of you hurting yourself when you're relaxed, so remember to move slowly with full awareness and have a calm mind.

One of the great benefits of the yoga exercises is that they help you to release any pent-up tension that you might be holding in your muscles, letting it revert back to usable energy. Yoga is similar to acupuncture or shiatsu in that each asana stimulates different subtle points, helping to relieve potential blockages in your subtle energy channels. After the energy is freed, it's a good idea to relax and allow the energy to flow freely throughout your body.

CORPSE: COMPLETE RELAXATION ON YOUR BACK (FIGURE 3.47)

When practising asanas, let go of the cares and work of your day. Bring your full awareness to your practice. The corpse pose creates a relaxed focus for your body and mind.

When to do: at the beginning, middle and end of your asana practice – also, any time that you are feeling particularly tense or stressed out.

Benefits of the corpse

► *As you breathe in, you're bringing additional oxygen and subtle energy into your body. Each time you breathe out, a bit of tension is being released from your body.*

► *Releases any lactic acid that builds up in your muscles during your asana practice.*

► *Complete physical, mental and spiritual relaxation – results in a deep inner tuning to your higher Self.*

How to do the corpse pose

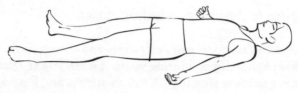

Figure 3.47 The corpse.

1 *Lie flat on your back. It's best not to use any cushions for your head, but if you have back problems, you may find that a rolled towel or cushion under each knee is helpful or to support your neck.*

2 *Bring your legs wide apart, at least 60 cm.*

3 *Let your feet and toes relax and 'fall' outward.*

4 *Have your arms out at a 45-degree (approximately) angle from your body.*

5 *Have your palms facing upwards. Allow your hands to relax with the fingers slightly curled.*

6 *Close your eyes (Figure 3.47).*

7 *Breathe gently through your nose. Keep your awareness on your breathing.*

8 *Breathe abdominally. As you inhale, feel your abdomen rise and push out. As you exhale, feel it fall and pull in. Don't strain or force your breath in any way.*

9 *To ensure that there is no tension in your body, you can shake out your shoulders and roll your head from side to side when you first lie down. Then bring your body to the centre and relax without any physical movement.*

10 *From time to time, you may want to check over your body to see if you can feel tension at any point. If you do find some tension, imagine that you're gently breathing it out with each exhalation.*

How long: remain in this position for 5 minutes before you begin your asana practice and for 5–10 minutes at the end. If you're relaxing between poses or groups of poses, be sure to relax until your heart returns to a slow, rhythmic beat.

Remember: to keep your eyes closed. Put your cares and other thoughts out of your mind during relaxation. Focus on your breathing for maximum benefit.

Caution: during pregnancy, it's best to substitute this pose with the Baby Krishna pose (see page 113).

RELAXING ON YOUR ABDOMEN (FIGURE 3.48)

When to do: between downward-facing poses.

Benefits of relaxing on your abdomen
▶ *Same as the corpse pose.*

How to do the relaxation on your abdomen

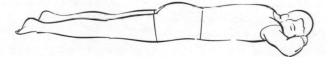

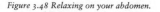

Figure 3.48 Relaxing on your abdomen.

1 *Lie face downward on your abdomen.*
2 *Make a pillow for your cheek by placing one hand on top of the other.*
3 *Turn your head to one side and rest one cheek on your hands.*
4 *Bring your toes together and allow your heels to separate (Figure 4.48).*

5 *Practise the same deep abdominal breathing that you did in the corpse pose.*

6 *As you inhale, feel your abdomen gently pushing into the ground.*

How long: remain in the position for 1–2 minutes between asanas where you're working face downwards.

Caution: don't practise during pregnancy.

CHILD'S POSE (FIGURE 3.49)

The child's pose is an important asana in its own right – and also a preliminary pose for the headstand and others.

When to do: between sitting poses, before and after the headstand.

Benefits of the child's pose
▶ *Relaxes your body physically and mentally.*
▶ *Prepares you for the headstand.*

How to do the child's pose

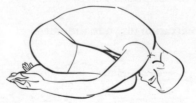

Figure 3.49 The child's pose.

1 *Sit on your heels in thunderbolt pose (page 64) and bring your forehead to the ground.*

2 *If your head doesn't easily come to the ground, or if there's any tension in your body when attempting this, place a cushion or block in front of your knees and allow your forehead to rest on it.*

3 *Have your hands, palms upwards, on the ground on either side of your feet (Figure 3.49).*
4 *Feel as though you're sinking down into the pose.*

How long: hold for 1–2 minutes.

Remember: there should be no tension in your hips or feet if this pose is performed correctly.

Caution: during pregnancy be sure to do the child's pose with your knees and legs apart.

BABY KRISHNA (FIGURE 3.50)

Although anyone may practise it, this side relaxation is especially good for pregnant women. You may want to add some cushions or bolsters to help support your body.

When to do: at the end of your practice session or between asanas where you find yourself lying on the ground.

Benefits of Baby Krishna
▸ *This is a luxurious side relaxation.*

How to do Baby Krishna

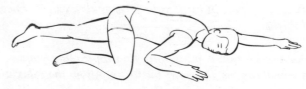

Figure 3.50 Baby Krishna.

1 *Lie on your left side.*
2 *Extend your left arm so that the upper part of this arm is acting as a cushion for your head.*

3 *Bend your right knee (the top one) and rest it on the floor in front of your body, or on a cushion. Your left leg (the bottom one) is extended with the knee straight, but relaxed.*
4 *Bend your right arm and rest it on a cushion or on the ground, tucked in next to your body (Figure 3.50).*

How long: hold for as long as you like.

Remember: your weight is on your knees, not on your abdomen.

FINAL RELAXATION

To obtain the maximum physical and mental benefit from your asana practice, treat yourself to a long and deep relaxation at the close of your session. Begin by coming into the corpse pose (page 109). Physically request that each part your body relax. Do this by tensing it and then letting go.

1 *Raise your right leg about 5 cm from the ground. Tense it and then let it drop back onto the ground. Repeat with your left leg, right arm, left arm – then with each part of your body: hips, chest and shoulders. Finish by slowly rolling your head from side to side once or twice, then bring it back to the centre.*
2 *Next, mentally relax your body. Without moving a muscle, begin by focusing on your toes. Feel them relax completely as a wave of relaxation begins to move up through your body, relaxing each part in turn: your feet, ankles, calves, knees and thighs.*

Feel the relaxation coming into your hips; relax your abdominal organs and your buttocks. Allow the relaxation to slowly move up your back. Let the muscles of your back relax completely. The ground is supporting you; there's no need to engage your muscles to hold your body up.

Feel the relaxation coming into your chest; your breathing becomes very gentle.

Relax your fingers, hands, wrists – and feel the relaxation moving up your arms to relax your shoulders and your neck. Experience the relaxation as it comes into your head to relax your face. Loosen your tongue and the muscles at the back of your throat. Relax your lips, chin, cheeks, eyes, eyebrows, forehead and scalp. Finally, relax your brain.

3 *After remaining in this pose for at least 10 minutes, feel the movement coming back into your body. Wiggle your fingers and toes. Stretch your arms up over your head – give your whole body a long luxurious stretch. Roll over onto one side and slowly sit up.*

You may want to follow your asana session with meditation (see Chapter 6).

10 THINGS TO REMEMBER

1   Before you begin to do asanas, relax for at least 5 minutes in
    the corpse pose. Also, end each session with about 10 minutes
    of complete relaxation.

2   If you have insomnia or frequent nightmares, you may find
    it helpful to go through the steps of the final relaxation
    at bedtime.

3   Remember to stand for a moment in tadasana before coming
    into any of the other standing poses.

4   Whenever you stretch your body in one direction, try to follow
    it with a counter-stretch in the opposite way.

5   Start from where you are. Your experiences and previous
    training make you distinct from everyone else. Try not to
    compare yourself with others. Yoga is non-competitive.

6   Come into each position slowly and gradually. Do not try to
    force your body to do anything that feels harmful or painful.

7   Breathe deeply as you hold each pose.

8   Backward bending is more vigorous and opens you up to
    new experiences. Forward bending is more introspective and
    calming by nature.

9   Most people start to lose the side-to-side mobility of their
    spines first – so don't forget to include one or more twisting
    poses in each asana session.

10 Smile and enjoy your practice.

4

Pranayama – working with breath

In this chapter you will learn:
- *what yoga breathing exercises are*
- *why it's important to breathe deeply and fully*
- *how to do alternate nostril breathing*
- *how to do kapalabhati.*

*Next comes pranayama which enables you to control the
flow of your breath and increase your vital energy. These
breathing exercises uncover the light of pure consciousness
and bring about mental clarity.*

Yoga Sutras of Patanjali, chapter 2, verses 49 and 52

Yogic breathing exercises are called 'pranayama'. The literal
translation of the Sanskrit word is 'control of the prana'. Prana
is the vital energy, or life force, that is known in Chinese as 'chi'
and Japanese 'ki'. It is the subtle energy that is manipulated in
acupuncture, shiatsu, reiki, tai chi and reflexology.

People, often unknowingly, use the power of prana in daily life.
When your child falls, you may rush over to 'kiss it better', thus
transferring prana. If your friend is sick, you may gently stroke his/
her head, thereby transmitting prana. When you bang your knee,
you instinctively hold your breath and place both of your hands on
the injury in an unconscious attempt to bring additional prana to
the area.

With regular practice, pranayama enables you to consciously manipulate the non-physical subtle energy within your own being. Pranayama enables you to cleanse and strengthen your physical body while calming your mind.

Why do pranayama?

Controlling your own mind is perhaps one of the most difficult things to do in life. After observing the intimate connection between the mind and the breath, ancient yogis came up with the idea of beginning by working with the breath.

If you watch a person who is at peace, engaged in deep thought or meditating, you will notice that his/her breath is slow and even; it may sometimes even be suspended for short periods. You have also probably noticed that when your mind is affected by negative emotions, your breathing tends to become fast, irregular and unsteady. These observations indicate the interdependence and interaction of breath and mind.

By its very nature your mind tends to be unsteady. It's constantly affected by the images it sees, hears and experiences through your senses. Pranayama helps you to make your mind one-pointed; stress is dispelled so that you can feel more peaceful.

Through the practice of pranayama your body becomes strong and healthy, your face shines and your voice becomes sweet and melodious. Regular practice of pranayama arouses inner spiritual force, which in turn brings you joy and peace of mind.

When breath is irregular, your mind is also unsteady. But when your breath is still, so is your mind, and you live long. Therefore practise breath control.

Hatha Yoga Pradipika, chapter 2, verse 2

USING YOUR BREATH TO DEAL WITH STRESS

Pranayama is the link between the mental and physical disciplines of yoga. While the action is physical, the effect is to make the mind calm, lucid and steady.

Swami Vishnu-devananda

How you breathe greatly affects your overall well-being in every way: mental, physical, psychological and emotional. Breathing gives you life. If you're not breathing deeply and fully, you may not be taking enough oxygen into your body to fully metabolize your food and eliminate toxins from your body. If, like most people, your breathing is shallow, you may be using no more than the top one-third of your lung capacity. If you keep your rib cage rigid rather than allowing it to expand with each in-breath, you probably find that you tire easily. Shallow breathing encourages you to feel stressed out and fall prey to frequent bouts of depression. When you walk around with hunched shoulders you cause vast amounts of tension to be blocked and to accumulate in your upper back and neck.

Watch yourself the next time you find yourself in a stressful situation, you'll probably notice that your breathing becomes even faster and shallower. But, instead of losing your temper or reaching for a cigarette or a drink, take a deep breath. The increase in oxygen intake will clear your mind and enable you to better deal with the situation.

By breathing fully you lay a firm foundation for your yoga practice. You will probably notice that the more deeply you breathe the calmer and more focused your life becomes.

Before you begin the actual pranayama exercises, it's important to make sure that you are breathing properly. Remember that inhalation is caused by your diaphragm moving downward. This creates a vacuum in your chest cavity, and air rushes in to fill the vacuum. Each time your diaphragm moves upward, it pushes the air out of your lungs, causing you to exhale.

Styles of breathing

DEEP ABDOMINAL BREATHING

Begin by lying flat on your back. Place one hand on your abdomen (just below your waist). Breathe deeply through your nose, taking long, slow, deep breaths. Feel your abdomen rise with each inhalation and fall with each exhalation. Be aware that you're making full use of your diaphragm. Try to draw the air into the lowest and largest portion of your lungs.

Practise this deep abdominal breathing for approximately 5 minutes before and after your yoga practice for maximum relaxation. Also, you may want to lie down and relax in this way between the various postures.

Insight

If you are having trouble breathing deeply, strengthen your abdominal muscles by doing this exercise with a few books on your abdomen. Breathe deeply so that the books rise as you inhale and then move downwards as you exhale. For a child with breathing problems, substitute a favourite stuffed animal for the books.

FULL YOGIC BREATHING

Be sure that you have perfected the deep abdominal breathing first. Then, sit up, preferably cross-legged on your yoga mat. If you have discomfort sitting this way, place a cushion or yoga block under your buttocks to relieve tension in your back and hips. Place one hand at the bottom of your rib cage. This is where your 'floating' ribs are located. They are moved by your intercostals, the muscles whose job it is to expand your ribs outward when you inhale and contract them when you exhale. The action of your intercostals gives your lungs much needed 'breathing space'.

Place your other hand on your abdomen. Ensure that this area
is also expanding as you inhale and contracting as you exhale
(Figure 4.1).

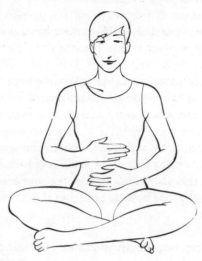

Figure 4.1 Full yogic breathing.

Visualize your lungs as long, skinny balloons. Usually when you try
to blow up a balloon, the part near your mouth expands, but the
lower parts remain empty and limp. As you take a deep breath, feel
as though you're filling up the bottom of the balloons first, then
the middle and finally the top. As you inhale, feel your abdomen
expand, then your rib cage and finally your upper lung. As you
exhale, feel this process reverse. Use your hands to check that
you're breathing fully and evenly.

You may have to practise this full yogic breathing for a few days,
even weeks, before you have mastered it. However, it's well worth
the effort.

It's suggested that you don't move on to the other breathing
exercises until you're able to breathe deeply and fully. If you're
new to breathing exercises, it's suggested that you next learn the
alternate nostril breathing before attempting kapalabhati.

ALTERNATE NOSTRIL BREATHING: USING YOUR BREATH TO BALANCE YOUR ENERGIES

Alternate nostril breathing equalizes the flow of your breath. It helps to calm your mind, releases stress and prepares your mind for meditation. Regular practice purifies your physical as well as your subtle body.

Before beginning to practise, try the following experiment: hold your hand under one of your nostrils and breathe out. Then hold the hand under your other nostril and breathe out. You will probably notice that your breath is stronger on one side than on the other. In a healthy person, the breath changes sides every 1.5–2 hours. As the right side of the body is controlled by the left side of the brain, this also indicates that the predominance of brain activity shifts regularly. The only time that the breath is even is during meditation.

In order to balance your breath and calm your mind, yoga students practise anuloma viloma, also known as alternate nostril breathing.

Insight
If you are having trouble doing these breathing exercises because your nose is blocked, it is best to start with some nasal cleansing (see page 129) followed by kapalabhati (see page 128).

Preliminary practice 1 – single nostril breathing
1 *Close your right nostril using your right thumb. Inhale deeply through your left nostril to the count of 4; exhale to a count of 8. Practise this, making sure that you're using a full yogic breath, 10 times through your left nostril (Figure 4.2a).*
2 *Next, repeat this exercise through your right nostril. Close your left nostril, using the ring and little fingers of your right hand (Figure 4.2b). Repeat the full yogic breath 10 times through your right nostril – inhale to a count of 4 and exhale to a count of 8.*

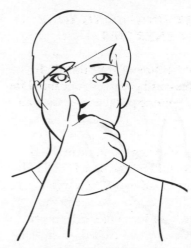

Figure 4.2a Single nostril breathing through the left nostril.

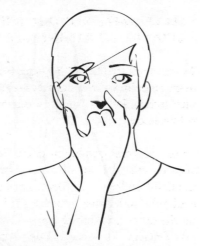

Figure 4.2b Single nostril breathing through the right nostril.

> **Insight**
>
> As it is more difficult to exhale completely than to inhale fully, yoga breathing exercises always emphasize the exhalation. A longer exhalation helps to strengthen your respiratory system, cleanses your lungs and provides ample space for you to breathe in fresh oxygen-rich air.

Preliminary practice 2 – alternate nostril breathing, no retention

1 *Bring your right hand into the hand position known as 'vishnu mudra' (Figure 4.3). You can do this by folding your index and middle fingers into your palm. Use your thumb to close your right nostril and your two end fingers (ring and little fingers) to close your left nostril.*

2 *Begin the exercise by closing your right nostril with your thumb and inhaling through your left to a count of 4 (Figure 4.4).*

3 *Change sides and exhale through your right nostril to a count of 8 (Figure 4.5).*

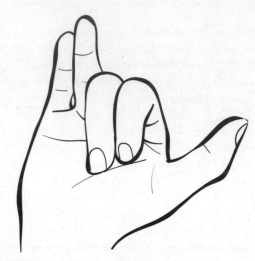

Figure 4.3 *Vishnu mudra.*

4 *Then inhale through your right nostril to a count of 4.*
5 *Change sides and exhale through your left nostril to a count of 8.*

Make sure that you're using the full yoga breath. Repeat this exercise 10 times daily, until you feel comfortable with it and are ready to take your practice to the next level.

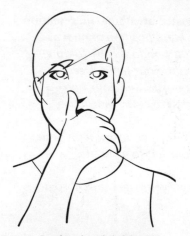

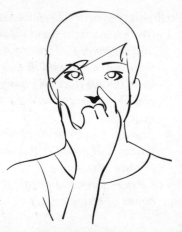

Figure 4.4 *Breathing through the left nostril.*   Figure 4.5 *Breathing through the right nostril.*

Preliminary practice 3 – alternate nostril breathing, half retention

1 *Bring your right hand into vishnu mudra (see Figure 4.3).
   Exhale completely through both nostrils.*
2 *Close the right nostril with your right thumb. Breathe in
   through your left nostril for a count of 4 (Figure 4.4).*
3 *Now pinch the left nostril closed as well, using your ring and
   little fingers. Hold your breath for a count of 8 (Figure 4.6).*
4 *Release your thumb from your right nostril and breathe out
   through the right for a count of 8, keeping your left nostril
   closed with your ring and little fingers (Figure 4.5).*
5 *With your left nostril remaining closed, breathe in through
   the right to a count of 4.*
6 *Close both nostrils and hold your breath to a count of 8.*
7 *Release your left nostril and breathe out through the left for a
   count of 8, keeping the right nostril closed with your thumb.*

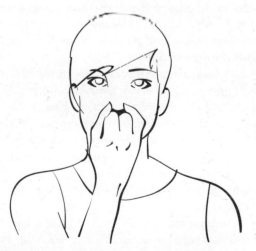

Figure 4.6 Retention.

Practise this exercise 10 times daily, until you feel ready to increase the retention time.

> **Insight**
> In all yoga breathing exercises, it is important to keep your back straight and fully upright. This frees your rib cage and gives it room to expand more fully.

Alternate nostril breathing with full retention
When to do: this is the full exercise that you can attempt once you've mastered the preliminary ones.

Once you've mastered this exercise, go on to learn kapalabhati.

Once you have learned both exercises, do the kapalabhati first, followed by alternate nostril breathing. Do both of these exercises before your asana or meditation practice.

Benefits of alternate nostril breathing with full retention
▶ *Your entire respiratory system is cleansed and strengthened. Stale air and waste products are expelled from your lungs.*
▶ *During retention, the rate of gaseous exchange in the lungs is increased as a result of the increase in pressure. This means that more oxygen from your lungs goes into your bloodstream. Also more carbon dioxide and other waste products from your blood pass into your lungs and are eliminated during exhalation.*
▶ *Your breath naturally alternates between the two nostrils, changing approximately every 2 hours. The breath in your right nostril is hot, symbolically referred to as the 'sun' or 'pingala'. It is catabolic (releases energy) and acceleratory to the organs of your body. The flow from the left, which is cool and referred to as the 'moon' or 'ida', is anabolic (accumulates energy) and inhibitory to the body. This alternate breathing exercise helps to bring equilibrium between the two.*
▶ *It helps to balance the hemispheres of your brain. It calms your mind, making it lucid, steady and ready for meditation.*

How to do alternate nostril breathing with full retention

1 *With your right hand in vishnu mudra (Figure 4.3), use your thumb to close the right nostril; exhale completely through the left.*

2 *Keeping the right nostril closed, breathe in through the left nostril to a count of 4 (Figure 4.4).*

3 *Pinch both of your nostrils closed; hold your breath for a count of 16 (four times as long as your inhalation – Figure 4.6).*

4 *Release your thumb from your right nostril and breathe out through the right for a count of 8 (twice the count of the inhalation), keeping your left nostril closed with your ring and little fingers (Figure 4.5).*

5 *With your left nostril remaining closed, breathe in through the right to a count of 4.*

6 *Close both nostrils and hold your breath for a count of 16 (Figure 4.6).*

7 *Release your left nostril and breathe out through the left for a count of 8, keeping the right nostril closed with your thumb (Figure 4.4).*

This completes one full round of the alternate nostril breathing.

How many/how long: try to do at least 10 rounds daily. You may increase the number of rounds gradually, if you wish. Also, as you become more advanced, the count may be increased, but always keep the same ratio of 1:4:2. This means that for every second you inhale, you retain your breath for four times as long and exhale for twice as long. Never change the ratio.

Remember: always use your right hand in vishnu mudra while practising alternate nostril breathing.

Caution: don't retain your breath if you're pregnant.

....

Insight

A gaseous exchange takes place in your lungs. As oxygen from the inhaled air passes into your bloodstream, it is

(Contd)

exchanged for carbon dioxide (gaseous waste products of cellular metabolism). You then breathe out the carbon dioxide. This exchange takes place at a slightly higher rate when you hold your breath for a short period, thus giving your body an increased burst of oxygen.

Kapalabhati: purifying the mind and body

The Sanskrit word 'kapala' means skull and 'bhati' means shining. In this exercise, you use your breath to cleanse your respiratory and circulatory systems. With regular practice, kapalabhati purifies your entire system so thoroughly that your face appears to shine with good health and inner radiance.

When to do: at the beginning of your practice session or before your meditation. Kapalabhati is usually done before the alternate nostril breathing.

Benefits of kapalabhati
▶ *Cleanses your nasal passage, lungs and entire respiratory system while strengthening and increasing your lung capacity.*
▶ *Helps to drain your sinuses and eliminate accumulated mucus.*
▶ *Eliminates carbon dioxide and other impurities from your bloodstream, permitting the red blood cells to carry more oxygen. The additional oxygen enriches your blood and aids the renewal of body tissues.*
▶ *The movement of your diaphragm and abdominal contractions massage your stomach, liver, spleen, heart and pancreas. Your abdominal muscles are strengthened. Digestion tends to improve.*
▶ *It refreshes and invigorates your mind. You feel an increase in alertness as a result of the increased intake of fresh oxygen. This often creates a feeling of exhilaration and an increase of mental clarity.*
▶ *It increases the supply of stored-up prana in your solar plexus region. This is your body's psychic 'battery'.*

How to do kapalabhati

Sit with your back straight and your head erect, preferably in a cross-legged position. Take 2–3 deep breaths, then inhale and begin the rhythmic abdominal pumping as follows:

1 *Contract your abdominal muscles quickly. This causes your diaphragm to move up into your thoracic cavity, emptying the air from your lungs and pushing it out through your nostrils.*
2 *Relax your abdominal muscles; passive inhalation takes place. Your lungs automatically inflate with air. Don't forcefully inhale.*
3 *Repeat this rapid pumping 20–25 times. End on an exhalation and then take 2–3 deep breaths to bring your breathing back to normal. This is 1 round of kapalabhati.*

How many/how long: start with 3 rounds of 20–25 pumpings each. Gradually increase this to a daily practice of 3–5 rounds of 30–50 pumpings each.

Remember: exhale as you contract your abdomen; allow your lungs to take in air as you relax your abdomen.

Caution: kapalabhati should not be practised during pregnancy. It is counter-indicative if you have a hernia, abdominal pain or cramping, or high blood pressure, or are experiencing an asthmatic attack.

As some people find the mechanics of kapalabhati a bit difficult to grasp, it's suggested that you initially learn it from a qualified teacher. Once you've mastered the basic concept, you're encouraged to practise regularly on your own.

Nasal cleansing exercises to enhance your breathing exercises

HOLD AND BLOW

1 *Exhale, and hold your breath as you gently pinch your nostrils closed.*

2 *With your mouth closed, imagine that you are trying to blow your nose.*

3 *Maintain a gentle pressure for about 5 seconds, with both your nose and mouth closed. This is similar to what many people do to relieve the pressure in their ears after their plane has landed.*

4 *Release your nostrils and very gently breathe in through your nose. Resume normal breathing.*

5 *Repeat this process 3–5 times. It may be practised daily.*

NETI – CLEANSING YOUR NASAL PASSAGES WITH A SALINE SOLUTION

Neti is an excellent means of cleansing your nasal passages and sinus cavities of pollution, dust, pollen and excess mucus. It is useful to everyone, and especially people with asthma, allergies and other respiratory problems. You can do this simple, hygienic practice daily.

You will need
- *a small 'neti pot' with a spout. These are available from most health foods shops, as well as many pharmacies and chemists.*
- *approximately 1 cup of lukewarm water*
- *½ teaspoon of fine sea salt.*

1 *Fill the neti pot with the lukewarm water. Stir in the salt until it is absorbed.*

2 *Leaning over a sink, breathe and hold your breath. Tighten the back of your throat as though you were about to gargle. Tilt your head to the left and pour the salt water into your right nostril. Allow gravity to drain the water out through your left nostril. Do not inhale the water.*

3 *Blow your nose and repeat the procedure by tilting your head to the right and pouring the water through your left nostril.*

4 *Blow your nose fully to eliminate all moisture. This exercise is most effective when followed by kapalabhati.*

5

Yoga lifestyle

In this chapter you will learn:
- *about the importance of balance in life*
- *how to act in relation to the outer world*
- *how to enhance your relationship with yourself*
- *what a yogic diet is*
- *how to fast.*

Yoga is not possible for a person who eats too much, nor for one who does not eat at all, nor for one who sleeps too much, nor for a person who is always wakeful.

Bhagavad Gita, chapter 6, verse 16

Moderation in all things

The lifestyle associated with yoga is one of simple living and high thinking. If you're a slave to your palate or have sold yourself to sleep, you'll probably find the practice of yoga difficult. Also, if you starve yourself or try to force yourself beyond your limits without enough rest, you will not find the inner peace of yoga.

When your external actions are in balance, your internal happiness seems to expand. Yoga is about moderation in all things at all times. You have to nourish your body and mind to have the strength to practise. You need to eat, but not overeat. Occasional fasting may be recommended, but not starving yourself.

Trying to expand your abilities doesn't mean forcing yourself into painful positions. Be gentle with yourself – but don't be too soft. Maintain a healthy equilibrium in all aspects of your life. Your speech should be measured, but say what you need to say. Don't be afraid to speak up.

Make a schedule; keep a practice diary (see Appendix 2). Leading a regulated, but not rigid, life helps you live gracefully. By providing material to satisfy your senses regularly, your mind remains contented – it doesn't get agitated easily. Yoga is the peace you experience when your mind is free from desires and yearnings. It's also the path that you took to reach that experience.

To be free from negative thoughts, try to cultivate the opposite positive attitude. But keep in mind that even thoughts that seem positive, when taken to an extreme, can disturb your practice.

Keeping your life in balance

Yoga is like a precious jewel with eight sides. It's a mystical road where you walk eight paths simultaneously. Asanas, pranayama and meditation are three of the paths of yoga, but the foundation is formed by the way you relate to other people and to yourself.

As you begin to practise asanas and pranayama, you will find your mind becoming more concentrated and probably more powerful. Without spiritual integrity and discipline, your new-found powers can put potent negative distractions into your path. If your mind is powerful, but bereft of ethics and morals, it can affect your own life, and that of others, in very negative ways.

Realizing the potential of this power to corrupt, the ancient yogis included lifestyle instructions in the teachings. These are designed to help you purify your mind and motives. Known as 'yamas' and 'niyamas', they include admonitions to practise truthfulness and non-violence; develop compassion; not to steal; not to be jealous;

and to learn to control your energy and cravings. Simplify your life; purify your mind and your environment; and try to be content. Continue to study; never think that you have 'mastered' yoga – and surrender your ego.

The yamas and niyamas form the foundation of yoga as a spiritual practice. If you live with and practise these values you will find your behaviour and thoughts moving in a very positive direction.

The yamas and niyamas are not harsh rules, but rather they form a living analysis of human potential. They offer boundaries and general guidelines for your practice. They suggest to you a way of living with more consciousness, integrity and joy. Their purpose is not to evoke fear of punishment. It's best if you can learn to respect these principles without moralizing or sinking into disciplinary attitudes.

Insight

If you would like to eliminate negative habits and thought patterns, it is best that you practise regularly. Don't expect instant results. At the same time you will need to introspect constantly. Look at yourself dispassionately. Try to witness your actions without making harsh judgements. Forgive yourself when you make mistakes, and then try again.

A WORD ABOUT KARMA

The Sanskrit word 'karma' has become a fashionable term that many people use with little understanding of its actual meaning. It means 'action', and every action has an equal and opposite reaction. Karma has nothing to do with your destiny or fate, or with being punished for your sins. The principle of karma is simple: if you throw a ball against a wall, it will rebound with a force equal to the strength you used to throw it. If you think of this in terms of your life, you will understand how your actions return to you.

Another way of summarizing karma would be: as you sow, so shall you reap. If you plant an apple seed, you will get an apple tree.

If you plant apple seeds, don't complain that you don't have any cherries.

In yoga, do your practice and reap the rewards. Don't resign yourself and think 'I won't do anything'. This is impossible. You can't not-do action – even for a second. If you're not doing something positive with your life, the lack of affirmative activity will result in negative consequences.

Take responsibility for your own actions. Don't blame others when things aren't going as you would like them to. You always have a choice, but sometimes it takes time for your actions to manifest themselves – so be patient, but keep at it.

You will probably find it helpful to take some time to understand the philosophical basis of yoga. Then, in addition to asanas and pranayama, begin to gradually incorporate these principles into practice in your own life.

Remember!
Success in your yoga practice is the result of six important qualifications:

1 *Cheerfulness*
2 *Perseverance*
3 *Courage*
4 *Knowledge gained from direct personal experience*
5 *Firm belief in the teachings*
6 *Solitude – time to reflect.*

Yamas – your relationship with the world

Your interaction with others should be in the spirit of the five universal disciplines: non-violence, truthfulness, non-stealing, continence and absence of greed.

Yoga Sutras, chapter 2, verse 30

Yoga gives you five 'yamas' or guidelines as to how you can best relate to the world around you. These are the boundaries and guidelines for your practice. They will help you to simplify your life so that you can be at peace with yourself and the outside world. They provide an ethical basis for social interaction.

Insight

Studying and attempting to practise the yamas guides you in developing non-violent sensitivity (ahimsa), honesty (satya), openness (asteya), healthy intimacy (brahmacharya) and generosity (aparigraha). These attitudes cannot be imposed upon you, nor can you develop them by merely imitating other people's behaviour.

AHIMSA

Ahimsa is non-violence. Refraining from injuring others in thought, word or deed transforms your aggressive nature and enables you to experience the oneness of all beings.

If there is a person with whom you are experiencing particular difficulties, use that person to practise ahimsa. Until you are able to love the person who injures or bothers you, it will be difficult to reach the deepest states of meditation. Your own negative feelings will always stand in your way

Ahimsa develops an attitude of reverence, benevolence and compassion for all beings, animate and inanimate. More than mere non-injury, ahimsa is positive, cosmic love that manifests itself as forgiveness.

You are expressing violence when you show contempt towards another person, entertain unreasonable dislike of or prejudice towards someone, frown at someone, verbally abuse or speak ill of someone, backbite or gossip, or ruin a person's reputation in any way.

Ahimsa is not cowardice; it is strength and wisdom. To practise ahimsa you sometimes have to put up with insults, rebukes, criticisms and even assaults. Also, be careful to not confuse non-violence with being passive. If you ignore violence and do nothing to actively try to stop it from taking place, you are a party to the violence.

First control your physical body. Then try to control your speech. Make a strong declaration: 'I will not speak any harsh words to anybody from this moment onward.'

Finally be aware of your thoughts. Negative thoughts can be far more dangerous than words and deeds. You harm others with thoughts of jealousy, envy and hatred. Greater than the harm you do to yourself with poor diet, drugs, alcohol and cigarettes, you hurt yourself with negative self-image, putting yourself down, neglecting your own basic needs – and even overdoing your physical yoga practice.

Some questions you can ask yourself in relation to the principle of ahimsa:

1 *Do I consciously hurt others? If not physically, am I in the habit of thinking harmful thoughts or saying hurtful things?*
2 *Do I impose negativity?*
3 *Do I tend to be judgemental?*
4 *Do I mask my fears and timidity with the pretext of being non-violent?*

Insight

Look at ways you may be harming yourself. Poor self-image may be at the root of the violence that you are unthinkingly directing against yourself by using drugs, alcohol and cigarettes, eating the wrong foods, or over-indulging in food. Overdoing physical practice, having negative thoughts about yourself, or making self-demeaning statements are also forms of violence that you may be practising against yourself.

SATYA

Satya is truthfulness, refraining from lying. Truthfulness is always accompanied by ahimsa (non-violence). It's important to express your vision of truth in a way that is not hurtful. Truth is not always easy to find, but searching for it strengthens your mind, integrity and inner resolve. Until you have released the 'baggage' that you carry, you will not be acting fully from satya.

The world is a relative place, but meditation and yoga practice help you to tune to the non-changing Truth. Unfortunately, most of us think that 'My experience is the truth'. There is a famous analogy in the yoga scriptures known as 'the poison and worms' that looks at how worms and bacteria thrive in an environment that would kill other beings. One person's poison is another's nectar. Good and bad are relative, but the highest Truth is not relative.

Tuning to the Truth involves constant analysis and checking of yourself and how you speak about things. Satya comes when your words coincide with your actions – and both words and actions are in tune with your thoughts – and an attitude of non-violence is present.

Some questions to ask yourself to understand your relationship to satya and how it relates to your yoga practice:

1 How willing am I to face unpleasant truths about myself?
2 Do I make promises that I know I can't keep?
3 How often do I try to avoid 'making a scene' by telling myself that I don't mind something when it really bothers me?
4 Do I allow myself to be talked into things that I really don't want to do?
5 Do I tell 'harmless' half-truths or bend the truth to serve my own purpose?

Insight

The great Indian yoga teacher Swami Vivekananda suggested that whenever you are undecided as to whether it is more important to be truthful or non-violent, it is usually best to try to not hurt others.

ASTEYA

Asteya is unflinching generosity of spirit. In the strictest sense, it means non-stealing, but there are many levels of stealing. If you're a teacher, be careful to not 'steal' your students' opportunity to understand for themselves by providing too much information. As a parent you may 'steal' your children's chances of becoming strong and free-spirited. It's possible to steal time, affection, space, credit/praise, ideas, energy, independence and free will, among other things. If you over-consume, you are stealing from the earth.

The commitment to non-stealing encourages you to not be passive while someone steals your neighbour's car or embezzles money from your employer. Societies also have a responsibility to refrain from stealing. In all major decisions the Native Americans considered the impact of their choices on seven future generations. This indicates a remarkable tuning to the principle of asteya.

In your yoga practice, be careful not to be overly critical and compare yourself with others. You steal from yourself by feeling inadequate and wanting what others have in physical ability, beauty, youth or spiritual attainment.

When you move beyond the satisfaction of your needs to the fulfilment of your wants, you enter the realm of stealing. In your yoga practice, take time to be silent so that you can listen deeply to what your body, mind and soul truly need.

Some questions that you could ask yourself to enhance your understanding of asteya:

1 *Do I 'borrow' things (such as books) and then conveniently 'forget' to return them?*
2 *What demands do I make of people? Do I waste their time? Am I emotionally draining?*
3 *Are my home and lifestyle in accordance with my needs?*
4 *Do I deny myself joy by being too self-critical?*
5 *Do I deprive others of opportunities that might help them grow?*

BRAHMACHARYA

Brahmacharya is the abstaining from excessive indulgences that result in the wasting of your energy. Don't let your mind get stuck on sense objects, control yourself, resist the outward and downward pull of sensuality and transcend body consciousness.

You may have trouble relating to the simplistic interpretation of brahmacharya as celibacy. You can better understand brahmacharya by remembering that you don't have different 'types' of energy. Saying that you have sexual energy and other kinds of energy would be like classifying electricity as lamp electricity, refrigerator electricity, television electricity, etc. In reality, the energy is the same; you can choose to use that energy for various purposes. If you practise yoga and your mind has become very powerful, using your energy purely for your own sexual and sensual enjoyment could prove dangerous. Perhaps this is the cause of the many scandals surrounding various spiritual organizations, with leaders being accused of misuse of the power that they have gained through their spiritual practices.

Brahmacharya is the art of self-control. You can see it as nurturing a healthy respect for yourself and your partner. It is refraining from meaningless sexual encounters that drain your energy.

A person who is a glutton or epicurean is not practising brahmacharya, even if they are abstaining from overt sexual activity. Neither is a person with 'diarrhoea of the tongue', who wastes much time and energy in needless talk and gossip. Through your yoga practice, you learn to control your energy and channel it in a positive way. What you consider 'positive' is your decision.

Relate the following questions regarding brahmacharya to your yoga practice:

1 *Do I waste potentially creative energies on excessive indulgences? Or on thoughts of them?*
2 *Do I waste the energy of others?*
3 *How could I apply the principle of brahmacharya to my life?*

Insight

By practising brahmacharya you create a harmonious relationship between the different manifestations of energy in your body: emotional, sensual, sexual, physical and the more subtle levels of thought.

APARIGRAHA

Aparigraha is the experience of fullness and abundance. If you feel complete within yourself, there is nothing for you to need or want. Aparigraha is often translated as non-greed, or refraining from the acceptance of bribes; not being overly possessive.

You may sometimes think that you need something to make your life complete. If you could have a new car, or a better job, or the perfect boyfriend, you think you would be happy. By gathering possessions and investing them with emotional meaning, you may be starving yourself of what you most need, i.e. authentic deep relationships.

Even in your yoga practice, you may be indulging in a subtle form of grasping, thinking you would be happy if only you could master some new fancy pretzel-shaped asana! You may be practising what looks like yoga, but for the wrong reasons.

Aparigraha warns against accepting hospitality or gifts with 'strings attached'. The purpose of yoga practice is to free you from the bonds of your mind. When you accept a bribe, even an emotional one, you are no longer free.

Here are some questions relating to aparigraha and how it may relate to your yoga practice:

1 *How attached/detached am I to my possessions?*
    a *Do I resent having to share things/space with others?*
    b *Do I hoard things that I'll probably never use?*
    c *Is my house cluttered?*
2 *Do I judge people by the things they have collected?*
3 *Do I surround myself with things that will enhance people's opinion of me?*
4 *Am I greedy for sensations and/or experiences?*
5 *Am I a control freak?*
6 *How can I simplify my life?*

Insight

Be aware of your attitude in your relationships with others – do you tend to always give or always take – or do you enjoy a healthy balance, as the situation requires. The true spirit of aparigraha involves deep generosity – not making notes in your energetic account book.

Niyamas – your relationship with yourself

In your relationship with yourself observe the five internal disciplines of purity, contentment, austerity, self-study and surrender to the Divine.

Yoga Sutras, chapter 2, verse 32

While acknowledging the importance of your relationship with others and with your surroundings, the ancient yogis also graciously left guidelines to help you to positively control your instincts and emotions. These 'niyamas' are constructive ways for you, as a yoga practitioner, to analyze your relationship with yourself. They extol you to view your body with respect without sinking into a moralizing or disciplinary attitude.

The niyamas are five personal principles relating to self-discipline. They advocate that you take positive action in taking responsibility for your own life. You will probably find that all of these principles are very much interdependent on each other.

Rather than telling yourself what not to do, they advise that you try to cultivate the opposite. You could put this suggestion into action when you want to get rid of some negative habit or addiction. For example, if you have wanted to stop smoking you may have noticed that it doesn't work to tell yourself 'I'm not going to smoke. No, I won't have a cigarette.' When telling yourself this you're actually focusing on smoking. Rather than focusing on the negative, it might be a better idea to begin a regular practice of pranayama.

Pay attention to one positive action at a time. Try to do it with full determination. When you repeat that action regularly, it becomes a habit. Build one positive habit at a time; see how they join together to form a happier and healthier lifestyle.

Insight

The niyamas enhance your self-responsibility, self-image and self-discipline. They are positive means of self-empowerment that encourage you to take responsibility for your own actions.

SAUCHA

The expression of the spirit increases in proportion to the development of the body and mind in which it is encased.

Swami Vishnu-devananda, *Complete Illustrated Book of Yoga*, page 19

Saucha signifies physical and mental purification. You create a pure environment for yourself: both internal and external.

Some people misunderstand yoga to be a 'cult of the body'. However, while yoga doesn't see the body as evil, neither does it glorify the body. Rather, it reminds you that your body is the vehicle of your soul. It's an instrument that works best when you keep it clean and strong. If your body breaks down, you won't reach your goal.

Saucha is purification on many levels. It includes the physical cleanliness of washing your body, maintaining an orderly home, eating healthy food and drinking clean water. It's also mental clarity as well as speech that refrains from emotionally charged obsessions and addictions. You try to find a balance in life that gives you a way to feel clear. As with the other yamas and niyamas, the practice of saucha enables you to enjoy the fullness of yoga.

Your physical body is purified by asanas, pranayama, cleansing exercises, a pure diet and fasting. Your mind and emotions are unclogged from psychological and sensory impurities through selfless service, meditation, positive thinking, philosophical enquiry and ongoing study.

Some questions to ask yourself to understand saucha:

1 *Are my intentions transparent?*
2 *What foods help my mind to feel clear and light?*
3 *What do my home and work area say about the state of my mind?*
4 *How can I cleanse my body, thoughts and emotions so that my true self can shine through?*

Insight

The reverence you bring to your daily life and the cleanliness you practise, when you are alone and in community, reinforces your sense of sacredness. The importance of the principle of saucha is revealed by the fact that Gandhi worked so hard at sanitation efforts in both South Africa and India.

SANTOSHA

Santosha is contentment. More than passive satisfaction, it's a state of mental awareness in which you appreciate the positive in all situations and in everyone with whom you have contact. It can be a dynamic and constructive attitude that can help you to view your life in a new light.

The principle of santosha helps you to be aware that it's your own mind and attitudes that 'cause' you to be happy or unhappy. For example: suppose you're sitting on a bus and suddenly someone puts their hands over your eyes. You may get angry or be frightened. If you turn around and see that it's a friend whom you haven't seen in a while, your anger would suddenly change to joy. Your happiness is not the result of what is happening to you, but of your attitude towards what is happening.

Santosh means being content in the present and striving to improve the future. Think how much time and energy you waste in reprimanding yourself for mistakes that you made last year, last week or yesterday. A vast portion of your energy is probably being consumed by thoughts of things that you shouldn't have done or that you should have done in a different way. Wouldn't it be better to learn from your mistakes and move on, rather than letting them devour you?

Through daily meditation and introspection, you can begin to intuitively understand that the past is past; you can't change it. Even one split second after you've done an action, you can't undo it. Once you've said something, it can never be unsaid.

You can't even change the present, that fleeting instant when the future becomes the past. By the time you realize what is happening, it has happened and is in the past. The understanding and practice of contentment can be a liberating experience. It can enable you to focus on positive improvements in your life and how you could best use your energies. By your present effort, you can change the future with increased vigour because your energy is not being drained by the past.

Remember that you have your unique gifts, challenges and ways of proceeding on your life's journey. Santosha is about being non-judgemental, letting go of constant comparisons, and accepting that you're exactly where you need to be at the moment.

Yoga philosophy speaks of the four sentinels who guard the domain of liberation. They are:

▶ *peace*
▶ *santosha – contentment*
▶ *wise company*
▶ *right inquiry.*

By encouraging yourself to befriend one of these guards, you find yourself in the company of all of them.

Ask yourself:

1 *How does contentment relate to smiling?*
2 *How does smiling relate to contentment?*

Insight

Santosha encourages your restless mind to give up its constant desires for new experiences, new tastes in food and new acquisitions that you may not need. Become aware of how your internal yearning consumes your energy slowly but surely.

TAPAS

Tapas is voluntary austerity that results in the ignition of a purifying inner flame. It is restraint of your mind and all of your senses. It means making your mind do something that it doesn't really want to do, or not letting it do something that it wants to do.

The purpose of tapas is to help you to purify and strengthen your mind. You do something that is difficult in order to develop your mental abilities.

If you wanted to make your arm muscles stronger, you might start lifting weights. If every day you lifted 1 kilogram 100 times, it would become easy enough for you to go on to 2 kilograms and gradually increase the amount of weight that you lift. You strengthen your muscles by giving them something to do that is a little difficult for them. You don't give them something that is so difficult that they can't do it.

Tapas is asking your mind to do something that is a little difficult in order to increase your mental strength and determination. For example, if you're a person who loves to talk, a powerful tapas might be to try to keep silent for one day each week. However, this may be one of the least appropriate tapas for a shy person. If you are timid by nature, it would be better to encourage yourself to speak up. Most people shy away from speaking in public. So, if you know that it's difficult for you, you could take this as tapas. If it's difficult to sing in public, then sing! You do it, not because you think that you're going to become a great singer, but because it's difficult for you to do.

For other people the austerity might have to do with food. Some people have trouble fasting, while for others the difficulty is eating. If you have an eating disorder, the most beneficial practice would probably be to eat a balanced, healthy diet.

Whatever weakness your mind has, tapas means trying to do the opposite. You try to do whatever is difficult for you, instead of glorifying your own weakness.

Tapas enables you to build up the inner strength to stick to non-violence. It gives you the inner zeal and steadfast attitude that makes compassion and forgiveness possible.

Try choosing something that you think you can't do – and make a determination that you're going to do it. It may be an asana that you're having trouble mastering, being cheerful for the week or anything else that you find difficult. At the end of the week ask yourself:

1 *How successful was I?*
2 *What did I learn?*
3 *What fears (if any) did I face this week?*
4 *What perceived limitation did I overcome? Was the limitation real or artificial and created by my mind?*

> **Insight**
>
> The practice of tapas is more than giving up a luxury. It means making your mind do something that it doesn't really want to do, or not letting it do something that it is inclined to do.

SWADHYAYA

Swadhyaya is self-study. Self-study can mean study by yourself, study of yourself, or study of the nature of the Self.

Studying by yourself can be reading about yoga – or it could be attending classes. This type of study is important as it gives you access to other people's experiences, as well as inspiration. Swadhyaya is not mere intellectual gathering of information.

For example, suppose you want to go to Inverness – you've heard of the place and, although you've no idea where it is, you just feel that you want to go there. If you just started walking, your chances of arriving in Inverness are slim. If you really want to get there, it's better to use a map and/or ask directions. The map and directions are the theory that gives you focus and inspiration. In your yoga practice, books such as this one will provide you with the necessary inspiration to begin and continue with your practice. It's important for you to understand the theory as well as doing the practice. If you only practise there's a good possibility that you will stray from the track.

The yoga traditions suggest that first you listen to a teacher, or read his/her book. Then think about what you have read or heard. Once you've intellectually understood the message, meditate on its inner meaning.

Swadhyaya can also mean study of your own mind. Sometimes, when you start your yoga practice, negative thoughts may arise. Even those negative thoughts can be useful if you're able to study them in a detached manner. Learn to be a 'silent witness', watch your own mind as though you're watching a film. Soon you'll begin to understand the nature of your own mind, and how to work with it in a positive way.

Appendix 2 contains a sample practice diary that you may want to use. You can pose various questions to better understand yourself and set goals for improvement. Taking it further lists some useful readings that you may want to incorporate into your weekly practice.

> **Insight**
>
> If you feel distracted and overly stressed, it is a good idea to include some regular study in your yoga practice. Swadhyaya enables you to understand the best way to proceed with your inner work.

ISHWARAPRANIDHANA

Ishwarapranidhana is dedicating yourself wholeheartedly to your practice and to finding peace in your life. It consists of letting go of your ego. We each have an ego; this is your sense of who you think you are. (Please note that the yoga definition of ego is quite different from that of Western psychology.) Your ego causes you to experience your physical self as being separate from your divine essence. As long as you have a body, your ego acts as a boundary that defines who you are. In order to have a universal, limitless experience you need to realize that all borders are mental creations that don't really exist. The purpose of yoga is to break down all boundaries and to help you to transcend all ego-limitations. Ishwarapranidhana is about becoming one with the Infinite. It is detaching yourself from your finite ego, and tuning yourself to the Infinite.

An analogy would be to take an 'empty' glass, which is really full of air. Think about the difference between the air in the glass and the air outside the glass. Really, there is no difference. If you want to join the two you have only to break the glass. Once the glass is broken, you understand that the separation was an illusion. Your ego is like the glass. When you get rid of the apparent limitations you realize that there is no difference between what is inside and what is outside. In the deepest states of meditation, your ego no longer exists. There is only an experience of absolute oneness.

The yogic diet

A yogic diet consists of pure foods that help to calm your mind and sharpen your intellect. Eat foods that soothe and nourish your body. A pure diet promotes physical health and much more. It encourages you to be cheerful and serene, and maintains your mental poise throughout the day. When you practise yoga, you're working on yourself on many levels.

Your yoga practice will be greatly enhanced by a simple nutritious vegetarian diet, occasional fasting and abstinence from negative habits such as smoking.

General guidelines for eating

▶ *Chew each mouthful slowly and thoroughly, remembering that digestion begins in your mouth.*
▶ *Pay attention to eating; savour your food. Don't eat while working at your computer, watching television or speaking on the phone.*
▶ *Try to cut down on snacking between meals.*
▶ *Don't overload your stomach. Fill half of your stomach with food, one quarter with liquid and leave the rest empty.*

- ▶ *Maintain a peaceful attitude during your meals. Don't argue over the dinner table.*
- ▶ *Try to have some of your meals in silence.*
- ▶ *If you're planning to change your diet, do it gradually.*
- ▶ *Give thanks before you start to eat.*
- ▶ *Eat to live; don't live to eat.*

THREE QUALITIES OF NATURE

Yoga philosophy identifies three qualities that are present in varying degrees in everything in the universe, including your physical body, mind and emotions. As part of your yoga practice, it's important to nourish yourself on all levels.

> **The foods that increase life, purity, strength, health, joy and cheerfulness, which are savoury and smell good, substantial and agreeable, are dear to the sattvic people.**
>
> Bhagavad Gita, chapter 17, verse 8

Sattva
Sattva is the quality of light, purity and knowledge. Try to make your diet as sattvic as possible by eating foods that are pure, wholesome and naturally delicious, without preservatives or artificial flavourings. A sattvic person is characterized by feelings of cheerfulness, peace and contentment.

When you eat sattvic foods, your body tends to be in a healthier state and your mind is free from excessive agitations. A sattvic diet includes foods such as fresh and dried fruits, pure fruit juices, whole grains, legumes, nuts, seeds, wholemeal bread, honey, fresh herbs and herbal teas, fresh vegetables and organic dairy products. A sattvic diet is easily digested and supplies you with the maximum amount of energy. It increases the vitality and endurance of your body. It gives you the strength to overcome fatigue, even when you need to do strenuous work.

If you are what you eat, your food preferences reflect your level of physical and mental purity. As you progress in your yoga practice, you'll probably notice that your diet is changing and your cravings for negative foods are lessening.

> *The foods that are bitter, sour, salty, excessively hot, pungent, dry and burning are liked by the rajasic and are productive of pain, grief and disease.*
>
> Bhagavad Gita, chapter 17, verse 9

Rajas

Rajas is the quality of passion, activity and non-stop motion. Rajasic foods cause your mind to be agitated. They over-stimulate your body, contributing to experiences of physical and mental stress. If you feel nervous and stressed out, try cutting down on the rajasic foods that you eat. They tend to destroy the delicate balance of your mind and body that is essential for happiness.

Rajasic foods include hot spicy food, onions, garlic, refined sugar, soft drinks, chocolate, processed and refined foods, foods that are full of chemicals and preservatives, coffee and tea.

> *The foods that are stale, tasteless, putrid, rotten and impure refuse, is the food liked by the tamasic people.*
>
> Bhagavad Gita, chapter 17, verse 10

Tamas

Tamas is the quality of ignorance, darkness and inertia. It often makes things appear other than what they are. Tamas induces heaviness, lethargy and laziness. Tamasic foods are stale, fermented, burned, barbecued, overcooked or reheated too many times. They include meat, fish, eggs, drugs, alcohol and tobacco.

A tamasic diet benefits neither your body nor your mind. It makes you feel dull, lacking in higher ideals and purpose in life, and devoid of motivation. Overeating is tamasic. If you suffer from chronic ailments and depression, try reducing the amount of tamas in your diet.

Non-violent diet

In keeping with the principle of ahimsa (non-violence) most practising yogis tend towards a vegetarian diet. Even if you have not personally killed the animal, you participate in the killing of it when you eat it. Adrenaline from the animal has gone into the meat and then into your system when you consume it. This causes disease in your physical body and a double injury has taken place. Not only have you killed the animal, but you have harmed yourself. Your body, mind and emotions are affected.

FASTING

Fasting can enhance the benefits of your yoga practice in many ways. When you voluntarily refrain from eating, you take advantage of one of nature's greatest healing agents. Fasting helps to restore your health and vigour. It often works when everything else has failed. Fasting gives your digestive system a rest, allowing your body to cleanse itself thoroughly. It removes waste matter, impurities that your body may have accumulated over many years.

Why fast?

- ▶ *When you fast, you don't have to spend time and energy to prepare and eat food. You are freer to focus on spiritual matters. All mystical traditions recommend fasting, often with vigil, as a means of strengthening meditation. In India, many people fast twice a month, on the eleventh day of each lunar fortnight.*
- ▶ *Even a one-day fast gives your body a rest; you feel lighter.*
- ▶ *As you lighten your body, your mind also lightens.*
- ▶ *It lowers ego defence mechanisms so that you are more open to divine inspiration.*
- ▶ *Fasting is a means of voluntary simplicity; a way to make your mind stronger and increase your willpower. Just as you strengthen your muscles by giving them work to do, you can also strengthen your mind by asking it to do something that is a bit difficult – like not eating.*
- ▶ *Fasting can help you to develop concentration and mental strength.*

- *Fasting prepares your body to absorb natural medicines. It also enables your body to absorb higher energy vibrations and be more fully conscious.*
- *Your whole system is cleansed and given an overhaul. During a fast, all of your energy that normally goes towards digesting your food is available for the repair and healing of your body.*

When to fast
Pick a time when you don't have to work, when you can be as quiet as possible, perhaps at the weekend.

Try fasting one day a week to maintain your good health and mental resolve. After a one-day fast you can return to a normal diet the next day. Two- to three-day fasts are recommended several times a year, especially at the change of seasons. Fasting gives your body a spring cleaning. Longer fasts of a week or more can give you great spiritual strength. After the third day, your hunger will disappear. If you would like to try a longer fast, it is advisable to have expert guidance.

How to fast
Fasting means abstinence from all food, both liquid and solid. Even juice is not taken during a total fast. Water is not a food. It does not stimulate your appetite and does not need to be digested. Drink plenty of water while you are fasting; it helps to cleanse your system.

Or you may prefer to undertake a juice fast. Although this seems easier than drinking only water, it is actually more difficult. The juice stimulates your digestion, so you become hungrier. However, it also stimulates the cleansing, so you may find a juice fast more beneficial. Try to take only fresh juices – either from fruits or vegetables. Dilute the juice with water. Do not eat solid food or fleshy fruits, such as bananas.

Helpful tips while fasting
- *Don't think about food and don't talk about diets.*
- *Use your time for quiet activity. Rest as much as possible. Try to have your focus inward.*
- *If possible, be alone or with other people who are also fasting.*

- Drink as much water as possible to flush out your system.
- Practise yoga asanas while you're fasting; this enhances the benefits of the fast as they enable you to eliminate toxins more quickly.
- Breathe deeply; pranayama enhances the cleansing process.
- Keep your body warm.
- Bathe frequently to relax your muscles and to assist the cleansing process.
- If you experience a headache or nausea, drink hot water with a little lemon juice.
- Avoid tea and coffee. Herbal teas, especially peppermint, are helpful.

Breaking your fast

How you break your fast is actually the most important part of your fast. Although you may develop food cravings, be careful to resist these impulses. It's best to begin eating slowly. Avoid heavy foods, such as milk, immediately after fasting.

On the first day, eat only raw or stewed fruits. These digest easily and help to gently restart the peristaltic action of your digestive system.

On the second day, add a meal of raw vegetable salad. This will act as a broom to sweep out toxins that have accumulated in your intestines.

In addition to the fruits and raw vegetables, include lightly steamed vegetables in your diet on the third day. Do not add salt or other seasonings to your food; enjoy their natural flavours.

On day four, add grains to your diet. Now that you have returned to a balanced diet, try to refrain from unhealthy habits such as coffee, tea, alcohol and meat.

Caution: don't attempt to fast if you're pregnant, if you have/had an eating disorder or if you suffer from anaemia. It's a good idea to consult your doctor or healthcare professional if you have any concerns.

10 THINGS TO REMEMBER

1 *The most important thing is to practise regularly.*

2 *People fail in their yoga practice because they overeat, waste energy by talking too much and don't persevere.*

3 *Remember that there will always be ups and downs in your practice. Some days you will be stiffer than others. Don't let this cause you to give up.*

4 *Be kind and gentle with yourself. But be determined.*

5 *Become aware of the effects of a healthy diet on your yoga practice – and on your life in general.*

6 *Cultivate a peaceful diet, as well as a healthy one.*

7 *Try to cultivate moderation in all things.*

8 *Simplify your life.*

9 *Purify your internal as well as external environment.*

10 *Watch your thoughts.*

6

Meditation – retraining your mind to let go

In this chapter you will learn:
- *what meditation is*
- *about the benefits of meditation*
- *practical principles for developing your meditation practice*
- *basic points of focus that you can use for meditation.*

Joy is within; meditate.

Swami Muktananda

What is meditation?

For many people, meditation may not seem to be an everyday experience. However, everyone, at some point in his/her life, has probably had some experience of meditation. It's a natural state, a universal experience – and an experience of universality. There's a good chance that you've already meditated without knowing you were doing it.

Think of a time when you were doing something that you really enjoyed. Everyone enjoys different things. Some people love music; others are mad about cooking or gardening. If you enjoy listening to music, sometimes you may listen for hours. When your mind is absorbed in the music you feel so peaceful that time seems not to exist. Or, perhaps you have had an experience where you became so engrossed in reading a book that you lost all awareness of the outside world. You didn't hear the phone ring or feel hungry when it was dinner time. You may have sat for hours without feeling tired.

You could say that at these times, you were in a state of consciousness that is very close to meditation. Your experience was probably a very happy and peaceful one, but your awareness was still in a state of 'duality'. This means that you experienced yourself as an individual, separate from everything else in the world. Although your mind was very concentrated, your mind was focused on something outside yourself.

Try to visualize your happy experience intensified many times. Imagine your mind becoming so one-pointed that there is no difference between yourself and your experience. Yoga philosophy sums this up by saying that when you are in the deepest state of meditation you experience yourself, the world around you and the act of knowing the world as one integral whole.

Meditation is an experience unlike any other. In it you go beyond the limits of your mind; your consciousness expands beyond time and space to a state of absolute oneness and complete peace. Yogis say that meditation is the experience of your own true nature. The Bible describes this state as 'the peace that passeth all understanding'. Meditation is an experience of the Infinite, which can't be understood intellectually or defined by your finite mind.

Insight

Meditation frees your mind from disturbing and distracting emotions, thoughts and desires. If you think you want to meditate but don't have the time, remind yourself about the benefits of meditation. It will probably cause you to work more efficiently, need less sleep, and to feel more relaxed and rested.

THE NATURE OF YOUR MIND

Your mind has its limits and is restless by nature. Most of us spend our lives being overwhelmed by one thought after another. A constant undercurrent of possibilities nibbles at your consciousness, giving you little inner peace.

In yoga philosophy, your mind is often compared to a lake or the ocean, which is made up of wave after wave. The waves seem to be changing the ocean. When the waves have subsided, the ocean returns to its tranquil nature. Unfortunately, most of us identify with the waves rather than the ocean. We become so caught up in our thoughts that we forget the reality behind them.

Your mind may also be compared to a book, which is actually a collection of pieces of paper. If each page of the book were to be torn out and thrown away, there would no longer be a book. The book would cease to exist. In the same way, if each and every one of your thought waves were to be calmed, your mind would cease to exist. Your mind, however, wants to exist – and your mind is very powerful. It's much more powerful than you probably realize. Your conscious mind is like an iceberg with huge hidden potentials deep below the surface.

If you're like most people, your mind jumps approximately a thousand times each second. This constant movement wastes tremendous amounts of your mental energy. But, as you begin to practise meditation and your mind becomes more concentrated, much more of its power becomes available for you to use productively.

Another analogy for your mind might be to compare it to the scattered rays of the sun. When the rays are concentrated by a magnifying glass, they are powerful enough to start a fire. Meditation is like the magnifying glass. As you start to meditate, you begin to develop the ability to concentrate; you're able to tap into vast hidden mental resources.

Meditation is beyond concentration. However, the way to start meditating is to try to concentrate your mind. Concentration is 'how to' have the experience, but meditation is the experience itself. Meditation is an experience of absolute peace. It's the state in which your restless mind comes to rest and experiences only the Infinite in the Eternal Now.

Meditation is a healthy, dynamic, enlightening experience – not a static or passive inability to move. It's a process of expansion, a means of complete personal transformation.

Meditation is not:

▸ *daydreaming or building castles in the air*
▸ *thinking, contemplation or introspection*
▸ *relaxation or sleeping*
▸ *therapy*
▸ *self-hypnosis*
▸ *praying or communion (i.e. having a deep connection) with the divine.*
▸ *The goal of yoga is 'union' rather than mere communication.*

Insight

Yoga philosophy speaks about four states of consciousness: being awake, dreaming, deep sleep and meditation. Although most people experience the first three states daily, meditation is no less a natural condition.

Why meditate?

After defining meditation, the next logical question you might ask would be 'Why would I want to do it?' Asking 'Why should I want to meditate?' is like saying 'Why would I want to be happy?'

Everyone wants to be happy; it's natural. However, each of us has different things that we think will give us happiness. Most of us spend our lives looking for the right thing or the person that will make us happy.

You may, like most people, think that happiness comes from outside yourself, from some object acquired or some goal achieved. If you ask people 'What will make you happy?', most people will say something like 'winning the lottery'. However, studies of lottery winners have found that after one year, they are no happier than they were before they won the lottery. In fact, many of them are less happy – they're constantly bothered by people asking for money.

Although you may intellectually know that happiness comes from within, still you may think 'I can't see it, so let me look outside. Perhaps the bright lights will help me.' As long as you think that there's a possibility that something outside yourself can make you happy, you will continue to search for happiness in the wrong places. You may find that you're happy for a short time, but when the happiness wanes, you will probably go looking for some new pleasure that you hope will make you happy. Eventually, after searching for many years, perhaps lifetimes, you may begin to understand that your happiness really does lie within your own self.

No object outside yourself lasts and brings you lasting happiness. But through the practice of meditation, you find yourself beginning to understand that deep and lasting happiness comes from the stillness that is the result of your mind being free, even for a moment, from the incessant chatter of thoughts and desires. Meditation is the experience of joy and inner peace. With practice, meditation makes it possible to see what your life is really about, what really makes you happy. It gives you powerful tools to change the things that need changing, rather than merely wishing they were different. The simple techniques of meditation help you to cultivate mental stability, strength, clarity and openness.

Yoga parable: searching for happiness
 A man went to an ashram and saw his teacher sitting in the yard with a big pile of chillies in front of him. The teacher

*was eating one chilli after another; tears were running down
his face. He kept repeating, 'This is awful. This is terrible.'*

*When the man asked the teacher why he kept doing
something that obviously upset him so much, the teacher
replied that he was 'looking for the sweet one'.*

*Aren't we all looking for 'the sweet one' – the one thing that
would make us happy.*

Learning to meditate is a priority for anyone wanting to lead
a happy, centred life. Meditation works on the deepest levels,
enabling you to bring about profound physical, psychological,
emotional, intellectual and spiritual changes. By practising
meditation you are able to work on many levels simultaneously
and change your outlook on life. The process of learning to
meditate helps you to develop skills that enable you to deal with
life in a balanced, open-hearted way.

BENEFITS OF PRACTISING MEDITATION

▶ *Reduces levels of anxiety and stress; provides relief for many
  stress-related illnesses.*
▶ *Increases intuition and empathy.*
▶ *Enhances feelings of love, joy, patience and compassion –
  'opens' your heart.*
▶ *Enables a clearer focus of mind.*
▶ *Provides greater energy and stamina.*
▶ *You need less sleep, while feeling more rested.*
▶ *Releases body chemicals that promote healing.*
▶ *Alleviates feelings of loneliness, disconnection and isolation.*
▶ *Amplifies your powers of concentration.*
▶ *Dispels depression.*
▶ *Promotes inner resilience, creativity and mental flexibility.*
▶ *Helps you gain insights into the nature of your mind and how
  to deal with it.*
▶ *Your experience of inner peace becomes so deep that external
  circumstances cannot disturb it. You develop the capacity to
  be grounded and balanced in all conditions.*

- *Enhances your ability to live in the present moment – not long for the past or worry about the future.*
- *Enables appreciation of deeper purposes; life assumes spiritual dimensions.*
- *Aids your capacity to go beyond physical and mental pain.*
- *Enables you to understand and experience the inter-connectedness of all life.*
- *Provides more clarity in your daily life.*
- *Allows you access to inner stillness.*
- *Promotes self-empowerment.*
- *Enables you to overcome the noise of your busy mind.*
- *Encourages less reactive behaviour.*

The practicalities

WHERE TO MEDITATE

An experienced meditator may be able to meditate at any time in any place. But, if you are a beginner, it's important for you to have a peaceful practice area. You can either create your own personal meditation space at home – or you may prefer to find a group with whom you can practise.

To create your own space, allocate a room or a portion of a room, which you plan to use only for meditation. It's best if you can keep this area free from other activities. After a while, you'll be able to feel powerful, peaceful vibrations being built up. Any time you sit in your meditation area, its energizing energy will soothe you; you will find this of particular benefit at times when you might be feeling distressed or have a problem.

When preparing your meditation room/area, remember the following:

1 *Ensure the temperature is comfortable.*
2 *Ensure the room is well ventilated.*
3 *Keep lights low or off.*
4 *The area must be quiet, with no outside noises or distractions.*

Focal point

Create an altar or area of focus in your meditation space. Keep in mind that the real focal point is your inner awareness. The purpose of the physical point is to suggest peace when your mind feels restless; to stimulate positive energy when your mind is sluggish; and to inspire you to reach deeper states of consciousness.

Things you may want to include in your meditation area:

▶ *an image/images that you find inspiring*
▶ *incense*
▶ *candle or oil lamp*
▶ *meditation mat and/or cushion – the mat insulates your body; a cushion under your buttocks will help to keep your back straight*
▶ *fresh flowers.*

Your altar can be as simple or as complex as you like. It may be as basic as a low table covered with a clean cloth. Or you may choose to create a more personal altar containing various pictures and/or symbols that uplift your mind. Your focal point is a very personal thing that serves its purpose best when kept clean, pure and free from negative influences.

Pictures/images

If you find that deity pictures inspire you, place one or more of these pictures in your meditation area. If you have, or are attracted to, a specific spiritual teacher, you may choose to include a picture of that teacher on or near your focal point. The picture will serve to remind you of the teachings. Pictures of family and/or friends will probably tend to distract you from your meditation practice; it's usually best to not keep their photos there. However, if a person is sick or in need of special prayers, you may want to place a picture there temporarily.

Many people place statues on their altar. Others may choose to put a symbol, such as an 'OM' (see page 173), a cross or a star.

Or you may opt for a simple area with only a candle and some fresh flowers.

Light or candles
Light is a common symbol of spiritual enlightenment. You will probably find that lighting a candle or oil lamp when you start your meditation practice helps you to focus your mind.

Some people choose to keep a light burning in their meditation area at all times, as they find that it enhances the build-up of positive energy. This is not advisable if you have young children or pets in the house. Or you may prefer a light only when you sit for meditation. The act of lighting the candle or lamp helps to send a suggestion to your mind: now it's time to be centred and tune to the inner light.

Incense
Sandalwood and frankincense have the effect of calming and centring your mind. The Indian tradition uses sandalwood whereas churches use frankincense. Scents such as rose, patchouli or jasmine stimulate the mind. They may smell very nice, but don't really calm your mind in preparation for meditation.

Insight
If you do not like incense, or feel that you are allergic to it, just don't use it. The burning of incense is not essential to your practice of meditation.

Rug, mat and cushions
Place a rug or mat on the ground in such a way that you feel comfortable facing your meditation table. It's usually best to face either the East or North side of the room as this enables you to take advantage of the favourable magnetic vibrations of the earth. However, this suggestion may be adapted to your living circumstances.

Have a cushion or yoga block ready to use, in case you need them to sit comfortably.

Meditating with a group

There are many yoga and meditation centres offering designated times for meditation practice. You may choose to join them rather than practice in your own home.

Meditating with like-minded people facilitates concentration as group energy is built up. You might even choose to start your own sangha (meditation group) for this purpose.

> *In meditation there is constant observation of the mind. It involves setting aside a regular time and place for the specific purpose of discovering that infinite well of wisdom which lies within.*
>
> Swami Vishnu-devananda, *Meditation and Mantras*, page 1

WHEN TO MEDITATE

If you lived a life in tune with nature, the most effective times for you to meditate would be dawn and dusk, when the atmosphere is charged with a particularly peaceful energy. However, modern lifestyle often makes it unfeasible to practise at dawn and/or at dusk. Instead, you will probably find that it is best to practise first thing in the morning or as your last activity of the day. Either one is perfectly fine; it's the regularity of time that's the important factor. To help you get the best out of your meditation consider the following points:

▶ *If you practise first thing in the morning, your mind will probably still be in a pure state. You haven't yet become involved with your work of the day. Or you may prefer to practise meditation as your last activity of the evening, when you can put aside all your cares of the day and take the opportunity to tune inward.*
▶ *Choose a time when you're not involved with daily activities and your mind is more apt to be calm. For example, if you have children that you have to get off to school, trying to practise in the morning might not be advisable.*
▶ *Try to meditate at the same time each day. Your mind will gradually come to associate this time with meditation, which will facilitate the practice itself.*

▸ *Before you begin, decide how long you will sit for meditation. Be determined that, no matter what, you will sit for this period of time. Begin with a 20–30 minute period.*

▸ *You will probably find that by meditating for half an hour daily you're able to face life with a peaceful mind and inner strength. Meditation is a powerful mental and nerve tonic. Divine energy flows freely during meditation, and exerts a strong influence on your mind, nerves and sense organs. It opens the door to intuitive knowledge and inner peace. Your mind becomes calm and steady.*

▸ *Try to not eat a large meal before you sit for meditation.*

▸ *If occasionally you miss your practice, be sure to practise the next day. Many people say 'I'll start again next week'. Don't put if off, start today.*

Remember: start right away; practise regularly!

WHAT TO WEAR

▸ *Loose comfortable clothing.*

▸ *You may prefer to keep separate clothing for meditation, as clothes hold vibrations. It's best to change out of your street clothes before you sit for meditation.*

▸ *A meditation shawl or blanket helps to contain the energy and insulates you from outside energies.*

Insight
Clothing made of cotton or other natural fibres is best. Jeans are not advisable, as they tend to prevent proper circulation (even when the jeans are loose).

How to sit

1 *Sit on a rug or mat, not on a bare floor.*
2 *Sit in a comfortable upright position, preferably in a simple cross-legged one (page 63). This pose helps you to steady your mind, and*

encourages concentration. It provides you with a firm
base and helps to contain the flow of energy, rather than
allowing it to escape. The classical lotus pose (page 66) is
not necessary.

3 *If you find that sitting cross-legged is painful, put some*
cushions under your buttocks to make sure that your back
is straight. It's important to make sure that your knees are
no higher than your hips. If your knees don't come down,
raise your buttocks up using a cushion(s) and/or foam
block(s).

4 *If you find sitting on the ground too uncomfortable, sit on a*
straight-backed chair. Place your feet flat on the ground in
front of you. Don't cross your legs or ankles. Do not lean
against the back of the chair.

5 *Ensure that your back and neck are straight, but not tense.*
This enables your energy to move up your spine unimpeded.

6 *Close your eyes and try to bring your attention inward.*

7 *Bring your hands into a position known as 'chin mudra' by*
joining the tips of your index fingers with the tips of your
thumbs. Allow the other fingers to relax (Figure 6.1). Place the
backs of your hands on your knees. Alternatively, bring your
hands together and let them rest gently in your lap. You may
choose to have the left hand on top of the right (Figure 6.2).
Alternatively, you may prefer to interlock your fingers
(Figure 6.3).

8 *Breathe through your nose, with your mouth closed.*
Consciously regulate your breathing. Begin by taking a few
deep breaths to bring a good supply of oxygen to your brain.
Then slow your breath down to an imperceptible rate. You
will find that your metabolism, brainwaves and breathing will
all slow down as your concentration deepens.

9 *Allow your breath to be rhythmic.*

10 *Your mind may jump around at first, but with continued*
practice, it will become quieter and more concentrated.
Don't try to force your mind to be still. This would create
tension, hindering your meditation. Be gentle, but firm with
your mind.

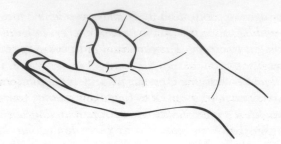

Figure 6.1 Chin Mudra.

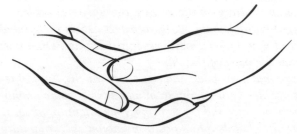

Figure 6.2 Hands together in lap – left on top.

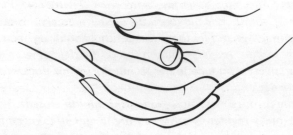

Figure 6.3 Hands together in lap – right on top.

11 *Select a physical area in your body on which you would like your mind to rest, like a bird on a perch. For beginners, it's usually best to use either the heart region or the centre of the forehead. The energy centre in the heart region is known as the 'anahata chakra'. The energy centre located between your eyebrows is called the 'ajna chakra', but is commonly referred to as the 'third eye'. We will speak more about the chakras on pages 176–178.*

12 *Begin and end with a prayer or inspirational saying.*

The clarity of your meditation tends to be greatly enhanced when you start with a prayer. Or you may feel that you're more drawn to poetry or an inspirational affirmation rather than to traditional religious prayer in your search for spiritual nourishment. It can be from whatever tradition you prefer. By beginning your practice in this way, you're tuning yourself to the divine energy. Sit down, say your prayer, make your resolve to sit for half an hour – and then begin your practice.

After you have finished your meditation, finish with a prayer, saying or poem. Then get up. If it's morning, go about your business feeling fully inspired. If it's evening, you will probably find that you fall asleep quickly, sleep better and wake up in the morning feeling fully refreshed.

Using your breath

Your breath, your most intimate companion, is with you throughout your life. It's the mediator between your body and your mind, responding instantly to your emotions and thoughts.

When you sit to meditate, one very common and excellent technique is to use your breath as your point of focus. This has a number of benefits, as your mind and breath are so closely connected. To see this relationship for yourself, you can try an experiment. Sit in a quiet room and place a clock on the far side. Sit quietly and try to count the ticks of the clock. You'll notice that the more you have to concentrate to hear the sound, the slower your breath will become.

If you have ever watched a cat trying to catch a bird, you will notice that she seems to not breathe at all. This is because, as we try to focus our minds, we all (even cats) instinctively slow our breaths.

Once you understand this relationship between your mind and your breath, you can use it to your advantage. Try the following meditation exercise.

MEDITATION EXERCISE: USING YOUR BREATH TO CALM YOUR MIND

1 *Sit in your chosen meditation position. See pages 166–168.*

2 *Be sure that your back is straight. Bring your hands into one of the positions shown on page 168.*

3 *Close your eyes and take a few deep breaths. Then let your breath come into whatever rhythm and depth feels comfortable. Notice how your breath rises and falls. Don't try to change or slow your breath, just watch it; be a silent observer.*

4 *Watch each part of your breath. Feel it on your upper lip; see how it enters your nostrils; feel it moving past the back of your throat, down your trachea (windpipe) and into the bronchi, entering your lungs and filling the air sacs.*

5 *Feel your breath halt for a moment. Then your inward breath turns around and becomes your out-breath. Watch the breath leaving your lungs, moving up past your throat, and out of your nostrils. Feel a bit of wind on your upper lip. Then notice how your breath stops for a moment, turns around – and the out-breath becomes the in-breath again.*

6 *Joyously draw in life with each inhalation and release pent-up emotions and impurities with each exhalation.*

7 *Feel the movement of your breath in your abdomen. Don't try to 'breathe'. Instead, allow the breath to happen. Allow the breath to breathe your body.*

8 *Watch your breath. Listen to your breath. Focus your mind and all of your senses on your breath. If your mind drifts off, bring it back to your breath. Your breath is your most natural focal point. It's also the universal obstacle to deep attention. As many times as your mind wanders, keep bringing it back to focus on your breath. With a bit of practice, your mind will come to this point automatically.*

9 *As your mind focuses on this point, cares and worries drop away. Visualize your mind being the water of a lake. When the lake is churned by waves, the water becomes murky. But when the wind and waves die down, the mud gradually settles and the water becomes clear. In a similar way, when your mind*

is freed from the incessant waves of distracting thoughts, it becomes lucid and clear.

How long: try to sit for at least 20–30 minutes daily, keeping your mind completely focused on your breath.

Insight

You may find listening to your breath more helpful than trying to watch it. Notice how when you inhale, your breath makes that natural sound of 'so' and as you exhale, it says 'hum'. You may use these sounds as your point of focus in meditation.

Focusing on sound

In the Beginning was the Word.

The Word was with God and the Word was God.

John, chapter 1, verse 14

For most people, it's easier to think of a sound than any other type of mental image. For example, you can probably 'hear' the Beatles singing 'Yellow Submarine' without much difficulty.

A particular taste or a certain scent wouldn't be as clear in your mind. Even holding onto a visual image tends to be more of a problem. If you try to visualize a flame, you might have some success in getting a general impression, but not an exact mental picture.

Sound doesn't usually shape-shift or morph as visual images tend to do. For example, try to picture a rose. You might begin with a red rose which then turns pink, then yellow. It begins as a bud, and then it starts to open, and then you see a garden of roses, and then you think of a time when someone sent you roses for your birthday – all kinds of associations arise. An exact visual image is usually more difficult for you to hold in your mind than an audio one.

For this reason, a common yoga practice is to focus on sound when you're trying to meditate.

MANTRA

A mantra is a sound with a positive energy. It's a word or a group of words, whose purpose is to bring your mind to a state of concentration. Mantra meditation is a path that leads you from the microcosm of your individual consciousness to the macrocosm of universal consciousness, using sound as your vehicle. A mantra is a mystical energy encased in a sound structure. When you use a mantra as your point of focus, the sound's energy is elicited and takes form.

The word 'mantra' comes from two Sanskrit roots, 'man' meaning mind and 'tra' meaning to take across; to free; to change form or change location – as in our English words transfer, transcend, transcribe, translate, transport and travel.

Mantras cannot be concocted or tailor-made for you, despite some current claims. They have always existed in a latent state as energies. Just as gravity was discovered but not invented by Newton, mantras were revealed to the ancient masters. They were codified in ancient scriptures and have been handed down from teacher to student for many years.

When you try to translate a mantra, it ceases to be a mantra because the sound vibrations created by the translation are different. The rhythmical vibrations of the Sanskrit syllables, when properly recited, help to regulate the often unsteady vibrations of your mind.

Meditating on the energy of a mantra takes your mind from the verbal level to the more subtle mental and telepathic states, and on to pure thought energy. This is a direct way of approaching the transcendental experience of meditation. With continued practice, the energy of the mantra has a positive effect on your mind and being. You may also mentally repeat a mantra when doing manual work or walking to catch a bus. When you repeat a mantra throughout the day, a positive energy begins to permeate all aspects of your life.

Meditation exercise: meditation on OM

OM is the original mantra. All other mantras exist in OM – the most abstract, highest mantra. There is no full, direct translation of 'OM'. It is the verbal representation of the transcendental sound that cannot be heard with your physical ears. OM is the manifested symbol of the original vibration by which the universe came into being – the yoga version of the Big Bang theory.

OM is a universal mantra which actually consists of three parts: A, U and M.

	A	**U**	**M**
Represents	Past	Present	Future
State	Waking state	Dream state	Deep sleep
Plane	Physical plane	Astral/mental plane	Beyond mind/ intellect
Sound made with	Mouth wide open	Mouth/lips rounding	Lips shut
Sound vibrates in	Abdomen	Chest	Head and sinuses

Chanting of 'OM' has a positive effect on your nervous system. It helps to awaken latent physical and mental powers.

1 *Sit in a comfortable meditation pose, preferably cross-legged. Make sure that it's a position that you can remain in without fidgeting for the allotted time of your meditation practice.*
2 *Bring your hands into chin mudra – join the tips of your thumbs and index fingers and rest the back of your hands on*

your respective knees. Alternately, join your hands together and rest them gently in your lap.

3 *Relax your shoulders and arms, but make sure that your back is straight.*

4 *Decide how long you will sit for meditation. Give yourself the mental suggestion that you will sit still and be fully focused for the next X minutes.*

5 *Offer your prayer or affirmation.*

6 *Close your eyes and begin chanting 'OM' out loud. As you chant it, make sure that the sound begins in the pit of your abdomen and moves up through your chest and throat, and finally into your head.*

7 *Begin with your mouth wide open – chanting the sound 'AAH'. Feel it vibrating and filling your entire abdominal region.*

8 *As the sound moves up, your mouth rounds to the sound of 'OU'. Feel it vibrating in your chest and then up into your throat.*

9 *Finally your mouth closes with a long 'MMM'. Enjoy the experience of the sound vibrating in your head, especially in your sinus cavities.*

10 *Continue chanting this elongated form of OM. Gradually make it softer and quieter, until you are whispering it – and finally repeating it mentally.*

11 *Keep your focus on OM, tuning it with your breath. As you inhale, mentally repeat OM – and repeat it again, tuning it to your out-breath.*

12 *If your mind drifts off, remember to keep bringing it back to the sound of OM.*

Other sound meditations

You may choose to practise meditation to help you to let go of negative tendencies and tensions. Take in joy. Experience the grace that arises in your mind after it has been purified through concerted effort.

Here are some suggestions to help you develop the ability to sit still long enough to concentrate your mind so that it becomes balanced, steady and one-pointed. When this concentration is intense enough and long enough, it develops into meditation. If your meditation is intense enough, you will move into a state of cosmic awareness – or bliss divine.

Steady and consistent practice is important – practise daily.

'Let go'

1 *Sit in a comfortable meditation position, preferably cross-legged. Sit on a cushion if necessary. There should be no stress on your back. Rest your hands on your thighs in chin mundra or bring them together in your lap.*
2 *Relax your arms and shoulders. Have your spine as vertical as possible. Your spine is your antenna to pick up and transmit cosmic frequencies.*
3 *Relax your face, with your eyes gently closed.*
4 *Give yourself the mental suggestion that you will sit still and be fully focused for the next X minutes. Try not to move a single muscle, or your mind will be drawn outward.*
5 *Offer your prayer or affirmation.*
6 *Close your eyes and bring your awareness to your breath. Give your mind something on which it can focus, so that negative thinking can be lessened.*
7 *As you inhale, hear your breath repeating the word 'Let'.*
8 *As you exhale, repeat 'go'.*
9 *Let go of expectations. Be still and open up to the experience.*
10 *With each exhalation, let go of pent-up tensions and aggressions. Inhale joy and energy.*

Centring prayer

In centring prayer you mentally repeat a word or a phase that you find particularly inspiring. Your word(s) express your intention to be in the divine presence. It's usually chosen during a period of prayer in which you ask to be inspired, with a word or phrase that is especially suitable. For example you might mentally repeat the phrase 'Thy will be done' or 'Have mercy on me' or you might use such words as Lord, Jesus, Abba, Father, Mother, Love, Peace or Shalom.

Centring prayer focuses your mind and inculcates the essence of the phrase into your spirit.

Repeat the same process as in the 'Let go' meditation but substitute the words with your own chosen ones.

Chakras – bringing your awareness to your higher energy centres

Your chakras are the interface between your physical and subtle bodies. Each of these seven whirling vortexes is the organizational centre for the reception, assimilation and expression of a certain type of energy, each associated with the qualities of a different 'element'.

Chakra meditations are simple, yet powerful techniques for helping you to develop your inner poise and keep your life in balance. The practices are most helpful when you reinforce them with a regular asana practice, self-analysis and positive activities throughout the day.

CHAKRA MEDITATION EXERCISE

1 *Sit in a comfortable meditation position with your back straight. Take 8–10 full, deep breaths. Then let your breath revert to its natural rhythm. Don't try to control it.*
2 *Begin your meditation by bringing your attention to the base of your spine, the region of your root chakra.*
3 *Gradually move your attention upward, visualizing each chakra as a flower that is opening in the sunlight. In the Indian tradition, the chakras are referred to as lotuses, but you may prefer to see them as another type of flower. Simply try to feel the energy of each chakra.*

With a bit of practice the energetic values of each centre will become clearer.

Muladhara: the Root Support
The first and lowest chakra is located at the base of your spine. Meditation on it brings you the gifts of its element 'earth'. It helps you to develop a grounded attitude towards life and steadiness of mind.

Swadhishthana: headquarters of Personal Creativity
Situated in your lower abdominal, sacral region; kidney, genital area. Meditation on the sacral chakra assists you in developing your creative impulses and the ability of its element 'water' to 'go with the flow'.

Manipura: the Power Base
Slightly above the naval in your solar plexus region, the third chakra controls the adaptation and transformational abilities that are associated with its element 'fire'.

Anahata: the Heart
Your fourth chakra is located in the region of your heart; this is the energetic centre of your body. Meditation on the heart chakra enhances compassion; its element is 'air'.

Vishuddha: the Communication Centre
Meditation on the fifth chakra, at your throat, develops your ability to overcome the limitations of its element 'space'. Your creativity and communication skills are enhanced.

Ajna: Seat of Wisdom
Focusing on the point between your eyebrows, meditation on the ajna chakra develops your intellectual and intuitive capacities. The 'third eye' is associated with your mind, which controls your senses.

Sahasrara: the 'Lotus of a Thousand Petals'
Your crown is your connection to the infinite. Meditation on this highest chakra goes beyond all elements and beyond your mind. It brings enlightenment.

4 At the end of your meditation, do a simple visualization exercise to ensure that you don't leave yourself too vulnerable and overly open to negative influences. Begin by returning your attention to the base of your spine. As you visualize the flower of the root chakra, see it closing its petals as flowers do in the evening.
5 Repeat this visualization with each chakra in turn.

> **Insight**
>
> Chakra meditations are simple, yet powerful techniques for helping you to develop inner poise and keep your life in balance. How smoothly your chakras function influences how fully you inhabit your physical body, the success of your relationships, and how much inner peace you are able to enjoy. By using chakra meditations you can keep your chakras open and operational.

Tratak – candle gazing

> *Look (without blinking the eyelids) at a minute object with your mind, concentrate until the tears come into the eyes. This is called 'trataka' by the gurus. By tratak, all diseases of the eye and sloth are removed. So it should be carefully preserved and kept as secret as a golden casket.*
>
> *Hatha Yoga Pradipika*, chapter 2, verse 31–2

Tratak or 'steady gazing' is a powerful meditation practice. You can practise it using any visual image that stands out strongly against its background. For example, your point of focus might be a black dot on a white wall or a white dot on a black background. Some yogis fix their gaze on the tip of their noses or turn their eyes upward to the space between their eyebrows. However, tratak is usually practised by staring at a candle without blinking.

When you prevent the natural reflex of blinking, your eyes will start to tear. This cleanses your eyes, tear ducts and sinuses.

Tratak meditation strengthens your physical eyes and the nerve centres in your forehead. It's also a powerful psychic cleanser of the ajna chakra, the 'third eye', and promotes intense concentration.

TRATAK MEDITATION EXERCISE

1 *Sit in a darkened room. Place a lit candle an arm's distance in front of your eyes. Make sure there's no draught so that the flame remains steady and non-flickering. It's best if your eyes and the candle flame are on the same horizontal plane.*

2 *Sit erect in a comfortable meditation position. Make sure that your spine is straight with your head erect and your body relaxed. Join your hands together loosely and let them rest comfortably in your lap.*

3 *Open your eyes wide and look at the flame with a steady gaze, trying to not blink. There should be no tension in your face or eye muscles as you do this. Hold the gaze for approximately 1 minute. Don't allow your eyes to cross. You will know that your eyes are losing their focus if multiple images start to appear.*

4 *Look deeply into the flame. Notice that it has several rings of differing colours.*

5 *After 1 minute, gently close your eyes. Relax your eye muscles and for the next minute, visualize the exact flame that you were just looking at. See it with your mind's eye. Hold it firmly at the point between your eyebrows.*

6 *You're not concentrating on the physical stimulation of the optic nerve that occurs any time that you look at a bright light. Instead, in tratak, you're using your mind to draw a mental picture of the flame, including all its rings and various colours. Hold the mental image of the candle at your ajna chakra for 1 minute.*

7 *Repeat this exercise, this time keeping your eyes open for 3 minutes, and then closing them for 3 minutes.*

How long: begin with 1 minute and then increase to 3. With practice, you may gradually increase the time to 5, even 10 minutes.

What to do if you tend to fall asleep when you try to meditate.

1 *Look at the time of day that you are trying to meditate; maybe you need to shift to a time when you are less likely to be tired. If it is an unusual tiredness, there may be some physical reason why you need to rest.*

2 *How are you sitting? Maybe you need extra cushions to keep your spine straight.*

3 *Check your posture; perhaps try varying your sitting position slightly.*

4 *Splash some cold water on your face; perhaps take a quick bath or shower.*

5 *Do a few rounds of kapalabhati and/or alternate nostril breathing, which quickly bring fresh oxygen to your brain.*

6 *Do a few rounds of sun salutation to wake up.*

7 *Make sure you are not lying down or sitting on a bed.*

8 *Don't feel guilty about falling asleep. The very fact that you are sitting to meditate is a sign that you are open to the experience.*

9 *Are you meditating after a meal? Digestion slows down your brainwaves and metabolism; it can make you feel heavy and lethargic.*

10 *Ensure that your meditation area is well ventilated.*

A FINAL WORD FROM THE AUTHOR

Reading about yoga and meditation can be fun. Interesting new books are released almost every week. But, to get the real benefit of yoga, you need to do three very important things: to practise, practise and practise!

Without practice, you become like a person who is starving while sitting next to food and reading cookery books. By practising yoga regularly, you can change your life in a very positive way.

I hope that the contents of this book will aid you in integrating a yoga regime into your daily life. May it bring great joy to you and to everyone you come into contact with.

I would like to finish with an ancient Sanskrit prayer 'Loka samastha Sukhino Bhavantu', meaning 'May the whole world attain peace and happiness'.

My best wishes are with you. May you enjoy great success in your yoga practice – and may you find great happiness in your life.

Swami Saradananda, 2007

Glossary

The following is a selection of terms used in this book, gathered here for quick reference. For more information, please refer to the relevant index entry

Ahamkara The ego; egoism

Ahimsa Non-violence, non-injury, mercy. One of the basic principles of yoga

Ajna Sixth chakra; centre of spiritual energy between the two eyebrows; the 'third eye'

Anahata Heart chakra

Ananda Bliss, joy, infinite happiness

Anga A limb, a part

Apana Downward-moving manifestation of prana

Aparigraha Non-receiving of gifts (bribes). One of the basic principles of yoga

Asana Posture, position, pose for meditation and/or body control

Ashtanga Eight-limbed; another name for raja yoga, as described by Patanjali

Asteya Non-covetousness; lack of jealousy. One of the basic principles of yoga

Bandha Lock; muscular locks applied by yogis during certain breathing exercises

Bhagavad Gita Literal translation: Song of God, one of the great scriptures of yoga

Bhajan Devotional singing

Bhakti Devotion

Brahmacharya Control of the sexual energy. One of the basic principles of yoga

Chakra The psychic energy centres, located in the sushumna, in the astral body

Chitta Sometimes it is used to mean the subconscious mind; at other times, it means 'consciousness' itself, or the stuff that makes up the mind

Devi Divinity in its female aspect

Dharma Righteous conduct; right action

Dhyana Meditation; seventh limb of raja yoga

Guna Quality or attribute; three qualities of Nature: sattva, rajas and tamas

Guru Teacher; one who removes darkness

Ida Left nadi

Ishwarapranidana Surrender of the ego. One of the basic principles of yoga

Jiva Individual soul with ego

Jnana Wisdom; knowledge

Jnana indriya Organ of knowledge; the five senses

Karma Action; the law of action and reaction, or cause and effect

Karma yoga Path of selfless service

Kirtan Singing of devotional songs

Kriya A cleansing or purification exercise

Kundalini Potential psychic energy; the primordial cosmic energy

Manas Mind; the thinking facility

Manipura chakra The third chakra, located at the solar plexus

Mantra Sacred syllable, word or set of words

Moksha Liberation; release; the term is particularly applied to the liberation from the bondage of karma, from the wheel of birth and death

Mouna Silence, a type of tapas (austerity)

Mudra (1) Energetic Seal. (2) Hatha yoga exercises, whose purpose is to seal the union of prana-apana. (3) Hand gestures

Muladhara chakra The first, lowest, centre of psychic energy, located at the base of the spine

Nadi Channel of energy in the subtle body, psychic current; the meridians of acupuncture

Niyama Your relationship with your self, including internal and external purification. This is the second limb or raja yoga

Pingala Right nadi

Prana Vital force; life energy; chi (Chinese); ki (Japanese)

Pranayama Control of prana, science of breath control. Fourth limb of raja yoga

Rajas Activity, passion, restlessness

Rajasic The quality of rajas, activity

Sadhana Spiritual practice

Sahasrara The thousand petal lotus; the highest psychic centre

Samadhi The super-conscious state

Samsara Continuous wheel of birth and death

Samskara Subtle impression; deep mental impression from past life; behavioural pattern

Sankalpa Imagination

Santosh Contentment; a basic principle of yoga

Satsang Association with spiritually minded people; company of wise people

Sattva The quality of purity

Satya Truth, truthfulness. One of the basic principles of yoga

Saucha Cleanliness, purity. One of the basic principles of yoga

Shanti Peace

Sushumna The central nadi, astral tube

Swadhisthana The second chakra, located in the mid-kidney/genital region

Swadhyaya Self-study; study of scriptures. One of the basic principles of yoga

Tamas The quality (guna) of darkness, inertia and infatuation

Tamasic Impure, rotten (with reference to food), lazy, dull

Tapas Austerities, voluntary simplicity. One of the basic principles of yoga

Vairagya Dispassion; perfect indifference to any object of desire of earthly life

Vedanta Literal meaning: 'end of the Vedas'. A philosophy of 'Oneness' based primarily on the Upanishads

Vedas The revealed scripture of India containing the Upanishads

Vikshepa Tossing of mind

Visuddha Fifth chakra, located at the throat

Viveka Discernment between what is permanent and impermanent/real and unreal

Vritti Thought wave; mental modification

Yama Ethics, restrictions; the first limb of raja yoga. Your relationship to the outer world

Yoga Union; discipline

Appendix 1:
Your yoga programme

Some suggested sessions for integrating yoga into your daily life.

Remember: start today!

30-minute practice

WORKING FROM THE TOP DOWN

1 *Sun salutation (tadasana)*
2 *Shoulderstand*
3 *Plough*
4 *Bridge*
5 *Fish*
6 *Seated forward bend*
7 *Inclined plane*
8 *Bow*
9 *Cobra*
10 *Simple spinal twist or spinal twist with one leg straight
    or half spinal twist*
11 *Tree*
12 *Final relaxation*

WORKING FROM BOTTOM UP

1 *Sun salutation (tadasana)*
2 *Triangle*
3 *Rotated triangle*
4 *Warrior 1 and/or warrior 2*
5 *Frog*
6 *Single-legged forward bend*

7 Fish
8 Upward-facing dog
9 Downward-facing dog
10 Reclining spinal twist
11 Final relaxation

60-minute practice

WORKING FROM THE TOP DOWN

1 Kapalabhati (tailor pose)
2 Alternate nostril breathing
3 Sun salutation (tadasana)
4 Dolphin
5 Headstand
6 Shoulderstand
7 Plough
8 Bridge
9 Fish
10 Seated forward bend
11 Single-legged forward bend or seated wide-angle forward bend
12 Cobra
13 Half-locust
14 Locust
15 Bow or boat
16 Butterfly
17 Kneeling crescent moon
18 Lion
19 Half-spinal twist or the sage's twist
20 Nataraja
21 Final relaxation

WORKING FROM THE BOTTOM UP

1 Kapalabhati (tailor pose)
2 Alternate nostril breathing

3 *Standing forward bend*
4 *Variations to the standing forward bend*
5 *Moon salutation*
6 *Chair*
7 *Cow's head*
8 *Cobra*
9 *Locust*
10 *Bow*
11 *Wheel and/or camel*
12 *Crow or peacock*
13 *Standing forward bend*
14 *Butterfly*
15 *Shoulderstand*
16 *Dolphin*
17 *Headstand (scorpion)*
18 *Final relaxation*

Appendix 2: Practice diary

Remember: don't say 'From tomorrow I will begin my practice'. 'Tomorrow' never comes.

Start your practice now and keep a diary to strengthen your resolve. Take a few minutes each night. The following is only a sample or suggestion. Write your own questions, in keeping with what you would like to achieve. Begin by writing your practice intention. For example: 'I'm going to do 30 minutes of asanas daily as well as 15 minutes of pranayama and 20 minutes of meditation. I'm going to cut down on my coffee/tea consumption.' Include in your diary whatever it is that you are focusing on in your practice.

If you didn't completely succeed in your practice intention, take some time at the end of the week to analyze why. Use this space to write down what you can do in the future to strengthen your resolve.

	Mon	Tues	Wed	Thurs	Fri	Sat	Sun
1 How long did I practise asana?							
2 How many sun salutations did I do?							
3 How much pranayama did I do?							
4 How long in meditation?							
5 How many cups of coffee/tea did I drink?							
6 Did I try to think and express myself in positive ways?							
7 Was I truthful?							
8 This week I am focusing on the following asana: How long did I spend trying to perfect it?							
9							
10							
11							
12							
13							
14							
15							

Appendix 3:
Schools and teachers

Finding a school

There are many styles of yoga; some are dynamic, others focus more on holding the poses. Some highlight the alignment of your body; others place more emphasis on relaxation, or on the co-ordination of breath and movement.

Many of the styles share common lineages. The founders of three major styles – Ashtanga, Iyengar and Viniyoga – were all students of Krishnamacharya, the teacher at the Mysore Palace in India. Three other styles, Integral, Satyananda and Sivananda, were created by disciples of the famous guru Swami Sivananda. This list is not meant as a recommendation of any particular style or teacher, nor to say that one style is better than another. Mostly, it's a matter of personal preference. It's a good idea to ask your teacher about his/her training and experience before signing up.

ANUSARA YOGA

Anusara (a-nu-sar-a) means 'to step into the current of Divine Will', 'following your heart', 'flowing with Grace', 'to move with the current of divine will'. It's a modern style developed by John Friend. Anusara yoga is described as heart-oriented, spiritually inspiring, yet grounded in a deep knowledge of outer and inner body alignment.

www.anusara.com
www.omshop.com

ASHTANGA VINYASA YOGA

The Ashtanga Vinyasa system is based on the system taught by the late Shri K. Pattabhi Jois of Mysore in India. Ashtanga can be physically challenging. Participants move through a series of flows, jumping from one posture to another to build strength, flexibility and stamina.

www.ayri.org
www.ashtanga.com
www.johnscottashtanga.co.uk

BIKRAM YOGA

This vigorous physical style of yoga was created by Bikram Choudhoury, 'yoga teacher to the stars' in his Los Angeles Yoga College of India. Bikram's classes are taught in a mirrored room heated to 95–105 degrees (so that the fascia, muscles, ligaments and tendons soften and stay more limber). Twenty-six postures are done twice each within 90 minutes. This is a vigorous, athletic style of yoga, designed to bring your body to maximum health and fitness.

www.bikramyoga.com
www.bikramyoga.co.uk

HATHA YOGA

Hatha yoga is a general term for the many physical styles of yoga. If a yoga instructor says he/she teaches 'hatha' yoga, it usually indicates that the teacher has learned techniques from more than one style of yoga and does not strictly adhere to any one style.

INTEGRAL YOGA

A gentle style of yoga based on the teachings of Swami Satchidananda, the man who taught the crowds at the original Woodstock Festival to chant 'OM'. The focus is to integrate body, mind and spirit through the combination of asanas, pranayama and meditation. Integral yoga was used by Dr Dean Ornish in his groundbreaking work on reversing heart disease.

www.yogaville.org
www.integral-yoga-centre.co.uk

IYENGAR YOGA

B.K.S. Iyengar developed his own approach to yoga over many years and has written numerous books on postures, breathing and yoga philosophy. The emphasis in the Iyengar system is on proper alignment – particularly for the spine and core of the body. 'Props', to help you get into postures or a modified version of them, are frequently used during classes. Classes tend to be moderately demanding; most classes end with a relaxation.

www.iyengar-yoga.com
www.iyengaryoga.org.uk

JIVAMUKTI YOGA

This method, created by David Life and Sharon Gannon, is a vigorously physical and intellectually stimulating practice leading to spiritual awareness. Classes are inspiring and fun, with a spiritual emphasis of the month and musical accompaniment.

www.jivamuktiyoga.com
www.jivamuktiyoga.co.uk

KRIYA YOGA

The system was brought to the West by Paramahansa Yoganananda, who wrote the famous book *Autobiography of a Yogi*. It's a relatively gentle, inward experience, not an athletic or aerobic practice.

www.yogananda-srf.org
csa-davis.org

www.ananda.org
www.kriya.org

KUNDALINI YOGA

Based on the teachings of Yogi Bhajan, a Sikh master, Kundalini yoga techniques focus on the controlled release of Kundalini energy through classic poses, co-ordination of breath and movement, and meditation.

www.kundaliniyoga.org
www.kundaliniyoga.org.uk

POWER YOGA

Teachers offering 'power yoga' are usually teaching their own modified version of Ashtanga Vinyasa yoga.

SATYANANDA YOGA

From the Bihar School of Yoga, based on the teachings of Swami Satyananda Saraswati, teachers teach asana, pranayama and relaxation (yoga nidra), and also teach chanting and meditation. Classes tend to be moderately physical to gentle. They have published many excellent books on yoga.

www.satyananda.net

SHADOW YOGA

Shadow yoga, founded by Shandor Remete, focuses on the progressive cultivation of the bandhas and development of the energetic body. It begins with a series of 'preludes', dynamic and rhythmical sequences combining warrior and sun forms that prepare you for the four levels of asana and pranayama.

www.islingtonyoga.com
www.shadowyoga.com

SIVANANDA YOGA

A moderate intensity, but challenging style, Sivananda yoga offers asana, pranayama and relaxation. Classes follow a set pattern of classical yoga postures; they emphasize proper diet, yogic lifestyle and meditation. Sivananda, one of the world's largest schools of yoga, was founded by Swami Vishnu-devananda and named after his teacher. Vishnu-devananda wrote one of the contemporary yoga classics, *The Complete Illustrated Book of Yoga*. First published in 1960, the book is still one of the best introductions to yoga available.

www.sivananda.org

VINIYOGA

Viniyoga is a gentle, moderate style developed by T.K.V. Desikachar, based on principles taught by renowned Shri T. Krishnamacharya. It aims to tailor yoga to individual needs so that yoga is relevant to every person and every situation. You will find a lot of gentle dynamic exercises – moving in and out of postures with focus on the breath. You may also find some meditation and possibly some chanting with the postures.

www.viniyoga.com
www.yogastudies.org

Finding a teacher

AUSTRALIA

International Yoga Teachers Association is actually based in Sydney and lists teachers throughout Australia.

www.iyta.org.au/contacts.html

The Yoga Teachers' Association of Australia (YTAA) is a resource and advocacy organization for yoga teachers.

www.yogateachers.asn.au

CANADA

Ascent magazine is published four times a year and includes extensive lists of yoga teachers throughout Canada.

www.ascentmagazine.com

Yoga Atlantic fosters high standards of yoga teachers, through a supportive teachers' network.

www.yogaatlantic.ca/teacher.html

Yoga in Canada

www.yogadirectorycanada.com

UK

British Wheel of Yoga is the largest yoga organization in the UK and works closely with the Sports Council. It promotes yoga classes, workshops and events for its members and the public.

www.bwy.org.uk

British Yoga Teachers' Association is a forward-thinking network of yoga teachers throughout the UK.

www.britishyogateachersassociation.org.uk

Scottish Yoga Teachers' Association, now known as 'Yoga Scotland' is a network of qualified, registered and insured teachers.

www.yogascotland.org.uk

The Yoga Register is an initiative created by the Independent Yoga Network (IYN) to provide Registration for Yoga Teachers and Yoga Teacher Training Schools.

www.theyogaregister.org/teachers/index.htm

www.yoga.co.uk is a comprehensive list of classes and teachers throughout the country.

USA

Yoga Alliance registers both individual yoga teachers and yoga teacher training programmes (schools) who have complied with minimum educational standards established by the organization.

www.yogaalliance.org/teacher_search.cfm

Yoga Journal is the largest and most popular yoga magazine.

www.yogajournal.com/OnlineDirectory

Taking it further

Asanas and pranayama

Desikachar, T.K.V. *Heart of Yoga: developing a personal practice* (New York: Inner Traditions, 1999). A modern classic, a simple, unpretentious insight into yoga.

Gannon, S. and Life, D. *Jivamukti Yoga: practices for liberating body and soul* (New York: Ballantine Books, 2002). A book to help you strengthen and deepen your practice.

Iyengar, B.K.S. *Light on Yoga* (New York: Schocken Books, 1996). The classic book by the internationally celebrated yoga master.

Kraftsow, G. *Yoga for Wellness* (London: Arkana, 1999). One of America's top teachers on the holistic nature of the practice of yoga.

Pattabhi, Sri K. *Yoga Mala* (Jois, New York: North Point Press, 2002). The world-renowned master of yoga lays the groundwork himself.

Saradananda, Swami *The Power of Breath* (London: Duncan Baird Publishing, 2009). Covers a variety of breathing techniques in yoga tradition.

Sivananda Yoga Centre *Yoga Mind and Body* (London: Dorling Kindersley, 1999). A positive guide to improved health, happiness and spiritual well-being.

Schiffman, E. *Moving into Stillness* (New York: Simon and Schuster, 1997). Yoga's secrets of stillness and movement.

Scott, J.C. *Ashtanga Yoga* (New York: Three Rivers Press, 2001). An easy-to-use guide featuring colour photographs and a series of step-by-step exercise sessions.

Swenson, D. *Ashtanga Yoga* (New York: Ashtanga Yoga Productions, 2000). Clear and concise with great pictures.

Vishnudevananda, Swami *Complete Illustrated Book of Yoga* (New York: Crown Publications, 1995). Offers a complete training programme.

Meditation

Long, B. *Meditation: a Foundation Course* (London: Barry Long Books, 2001). Ten concise lessons, complete with simple exercises that you can use in daily life.

Muktananda, Swami *Meditate: Happiness Lies Within You* (New York: Siddha Yoga Publication, 1999). Practical and philosophical teachings on meditation, like a short course in meditation.

Sivananda Yoga Vedanta Centre *The Sivananda Book of Meditation* (London: Gaia Books, 2003). A book geared to beginners and to those already experienced in the art of meditation.

Vishnu-devananda, Swami *Meditation and Mantras* (New York; OM Lotus Publishing, 1978). A comprehensive sourcebook of meditation, mantras and other techniques of self-inquiry.

Anatomy

Jarmey, C. *The Anatomy of Yoga* (West Sussex: Lotus Publishing, 2007). A full-colour illustrated reference book detailing the actions of skeletal muscles in over 100 yoga asanas.

Kaminoff, L. *Yoga Anatomy* (Leeds: Human Kinetics Europe Ltd, 2007). Detailed anatomical illustrations of all standard yoga poses used by the majority of yoga practices.

Mantras and Sound

Ashley-Farrand, T. *Healing Mantras: Using Sound Affirmations for Personal Power, Creativity and Healing* (New York: Ballantine Publishing, 1991). A practical guide that makes the strengths and benefits of mantras available to everyone.

Chakras

Johari, H. *Chakras: Energy Centers of Transformation* (Vermont: Destiny Books, 2000). Classic principles of the chakras.

Saradananda, Swami *Chakra Meditation* (London: Duncan Baird Publishing, 2008). By the author of *Relax and Unwind with Yoga*; theoretical understanding plus practical applications.

Saradananda, Swami *The Essential Guide to Chakras* (London: Duncan Baird Publishing, 2011).

Diet

Sivananda Yoga Vedanta Centre *The Yoga Cookbook* (London: Gaia Books, 1999). A vegetarian cookbook filled with delicious recipes in keeping with yoga philosophy.

Miscellaneous

Cope, S. *The Wisdom of Yoga*; (New York: Bantam Dell, 2006). An irreverent yet profound guide to the most sophisticated teachings of the yoga wisdom tradition.

Feuerstein, G. *The Yoga Tradition: its History, Literature, Philosophy and Practice* (Arizona: Hohm Press 1998). A unique reference work.

Sivananda, Swami *Bhagavad Gita* (Rishikesh, India, Divine Life Society 1942).

Vishnu-devananda, Swami *Hatha Yoga Pradipika* (New York: OM Lotus Publishing 1987). The ancient scripture of hatha yoga with direct translation and modern commentary.

Zambito, Salvatore *The Unadorned Thread of Yoga* (Poulsbo, WA: The Yoga Sutra Institute, 1992). An excellent compilation of translations of Patanjali's Yoga Sutras.

The author, Swami Saradananda, may be contacted through her website: www.flyingmountainyoga.org

Index